Global Perspectives on Palliative Care

Edited by Karen Bullock

Published in London, United Kingdom

Global Perspectives on Palliative Care
http://dx.doi.org/10.5772/intechopen.1005946
Edited by Karen Bullock

Contributors
Adhari Al Zaabi, Amna Al-Harrasi, Angèle Hermine Pondy Ongotsoyi, Atika AlMusalami, Audrey Miyehane, Constance Dahlin, Entesar AlYafai, Erna Haraldsdottir, Felix Fung-Yu Mak, Gloria Ka-Ming Chun, Jessica Curd, Kafayat Oyinlade Mahmoud, Laia Riera-Negre, Laura Murielle Kuate Makowa, Louise Loe Renee, Maria Rosa Rosselló, Mateja Lopuh, Nasr Al-Riyami, Nawal Al Mahyijari, Oyinlola Oluwagbemiga, Padma Sesha Sarada Lingaraju, Patience Tazanou Ngouanet, Purnima Jain, Rawan AlMujaini, Sebastià Verger, Sserusiba Hassan, Terrance Ruth, Victoria Ka-Ying Hui, Vivian W. Q. Lou, Zhuyun Lin

First published in London, United Kingdom, 2025 by IntechOpen
IntechOpen is the global imprint of INTECHOPEN LIMITED, registered in England and Wales, registration number: 11086078, 167-169 Great Portland Street, London, W1W 5PF, United Kingdom

For EU product safety concerns: IN TECH d.o.o., Prolaz Marije Krucifikse Kozulić 3, 51000 Rijeka, Croatia, info@intechopen.com or visit our website at intechopen.com.

British Library Cataloguing-in-Publication Data
A catalogue record for this book is available from the British Library

Global Perspectives on Palliative Care
Edited by Karen Bullock
p. cm.
Print ISBN 978-1-83634-410-0
Online ISBN 978-1-83634-409-4
eBook (PDF) ISBN 978-1-83634-411-7

If disposing of this product, please recycle the paper responsibly.

Meet the editor

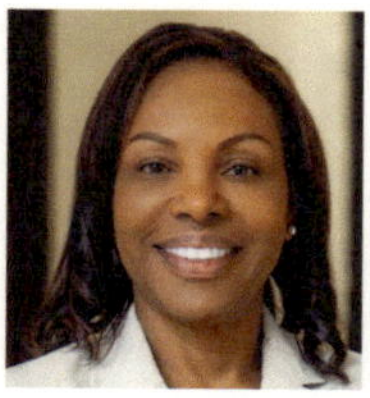

Dr. Bullock is an American medical sociologist, clinical social worker, and academic research scholar. She currently serves as the Louise McMahon Ahearn Endowed Professor of Social Work and has an appointment in Global Public Health at Boston College in Boston, Massachusetts (USA). She is chair of the National Association of Social Workers (NASW) National Committee on Racial and Ethnic Diversity (NCORED). Dr. Bullock is most known for her work on health equity, disparities, hospice, palliative and end-of-life care. She is a member of the National Academies of Sciences, Engineering, and Medicine Roundtable Committee on Quality Care for People with Serious Illness, and won the 2012 Best Article Award from the *Routledge Journal of Social Work in End-of-Life and Palliative Care.*

Contents

Preface

Global Perspectives on Palliative Care is a compilation of research reports, integrative literature reviews, case studies, and expert perspectives exploring palliative care through a global scope of practice. The book goes beyond the conventional frameworks and paradigms to offer strategies for improving equitable access to palliative care services across age and disease, focusing on often overlooked conditions, and it includes a humanitarian perspective. Each chapter concludes with recommendations for culturally competent practices. This book is designed for practitioners, educators, students, and researchers working in palliative, hospice, and end-of-life care. It is intended to guide practitioners in social work, nursing, medicine, pastoral care, and other health-related disciplines to understand the importance of cultural awareness, skills, and knowledge. All chapters are written by global researchers and edited by a leading expert in the field. Readers will gain a deep understanding from this vast array of work and innovation in serious illness care. The academic editor is thankful to all authors who have contributed their original work in this book.

Karen Bullock, PhD, LICSW, FGSA, APHSW-C
Boston College,
School of Social Work and Global Public Health,
Chestnut Hill, Massachusetts, USA

Section 1

Perspectives

Chapter 1

Perspective Chapter: Global Perspectives on Disability and Palliative Care

Jessica Curd

Abstract

This chapter explores the intersection of disability and palliative care from a global perspective, emphasizing the critical need to elevate the voices of dying persons, caregivers, and care organizations worldwide. It delves into the unique needs of dying individuals and caregivers with disabilities, a topic often overlooked in existing literature. Focusing particularly on people with intellectual and developmental disabilities (IDD), the chapter examines how marginalization is compounded by additional layers of race, culture, and socioeconomic status. In many Western cultures that are death-avoidant, these individuals face further marginalization. Drawing on Dr. Kimberlé Crenshaw's intersectionality framework and a critical disability justice lens, this chapter highlights the compounded injustices inflicted on marginalized persons, cultures, and communities. It advocates for a more inclusive and equitable approach to palliative care, calling for global contributions, collaboration, and change to ensure inclusive practices are implemented worldwide.

Keywords: disability, global, palliative care, hospice, intersectionality, equity

1. Introduction

The intersection of disability and palliative care is a critical area of study that has been largely overlooked in existing literature. This chapter aims to first share foundational definitions and concepts of palliative care and disability, building on these by exploring the unique needs of dying people with disabilities and their caregivers. Elevating voices of vulnerable people, such as people who are dying and people with disability, is essential for creating inclusive and equitable palliative care practices [1].

Disability, particularly intellectual and developmental disabilities (IDD), presents unique challenges in the context of palliative care. Individuals with IDD often face compounded marginalization due to stigma and misunderstanding about disability and also IDD, with some having additional layers of discrimination and exclusion due to race, culture, and socioeconomic status [2]. In many Western, death avoidant cultures, these individuals experience further marginalization, making it imperative to access and elevate their voices and meet their needs in palliative care settings [3].

Drawing on Dr. Kimberlé Crenshaw's intersectionality framework, this chapter highlights the compounded injustices inflicted on marginalized persons, cultures, and communities [4]. Intersectionality provides a lens through which we can understand how various forms of discrimination intersect and overlap to create new constellations of identity and marginalization which can exacerbate the challenges faced by individuals with disabilities at the end of life [5]. By adopting a critical disability justice lens, we can advocate for a more inclusive and equitable approach to palliative care that recognizes, centers, and addresses these compounded injustices [6].

The objectives of this chapter are to examine the intersection of disability and palliative care, identify the unique needs of dying people with disabilities, and propose strategies for creating inclusive and equitable palliative care practices. By focusing on global contributions and collaboration, this chapter aims to ensure that inclusive practices are informed by global perspectives and highlighting the need for global level learning and change. Recognizing the increased globalization, particularly since the advent of the worldwide web and social media platforms, it takes diverse perspectives and unity to achieve inclusion and quality of life for dying individuals with disabilities and their caregivers [7].

In summary, this chapter aims to explore and give voice to the experiences of dying individuals with disabilities and advocate for a more inclusive and equitable approach to palliative care. By improving our understanding of their unique needs and promoting global change, we can create a more just and inclusive palliative care system that provides quality and specialized care [8].

2. Disability and palliative care

2.1 Definition and scope of disability

Disability encompasses various physical, mental, and sensory challenges or conditions. According to the World Health Organization (WHO), disability is defined as an umbrella term for many different types of conditions that impact functioning in some way [9]. Disabilities can be congenital or acquired and may affect individuals' ability to perform daily activities and participate fully in society [10].

The scope of disability is broad, including conditions such as intellectual and developmental disabilities (IDD), physical disabilities, mental health conditions, and sensory related disabilities. Intellectual and developmental disabilities are characterized by significant limitations in intellectual functioning and adaptive behavior, which affect conceptual, social, and practical skills as well as social skills and communication [11]. Physical disabilities involve impairments in bodily functions or structures, while sensory disabilities affect vision, hearing, or other sensory functions [10]. Mental health-related disabilities impact mood, cognition, behavior, and potentially the level of social and emotional functioning as well [12].

2.2 Definition and overview of palliative care

Palliative care is a specialized medical approach aimed at improving the quality of life and comfort for individuals with chronic or serious illnesses. It focuses on providing relief from symptoms, pain, and stress, regardless of the diagnosis or stage of the disease [13]. The primary goal of palliative care is to enhance the well-being of both patients and their families by addressing physical, emotional, spiritual, and social needs [14]. End of life care not only focuses on preparing dying people and their families for death but in making meaning of these experiences and living as fully as possible until dying, with this care being important to end of life goals and wishes and equitable access being deeply important [15].

End of life care provided broadly and professionally is palliative care [16]. Palliative care is delivered by an interprofessional team of clinicians, including doctors, nurses, social workers, chaplains, and health aides [17]. This team works collaboratively to create personalized care plans that align with the patient's values, preferences, and needs [18]. Palliative care can be provided alongside curative treatments as well as radiation or other invasive procedures that may be used to ease pain and is appropriate for patients at any stage of a serious illness [13]. Palliative care is a larger umbrella for palliation of pain and symptoms, with hospice care being more a final stage of palliative care and also being interdisciplinary in approach [19].

2.3 Intersection of disability and palliative care

The intersection of disability and palliative care presents unique challenges and opportunities for improving the quality end of life for individuals with disabilities. People with disabilities, particularly those with intellectual and developmental disabilities, often face significant barriers to accessing palliative care services [11]. These barriers include a lack of awareness of IDD or how to market and educate to this population among healthcare providers and organizations, inadequate training in disability-specific needs, potential social or communication barriers for people with disabilities, and systemic healthcare inequalities [11]. They also include the general exclusion of people with IDD or their families in informing palliative care research or training [11, 19]. Moreover, people with IDD often experience social and physical isolation, even with community efforts in place to better promote inclusion, with older adults and people with disabilities already being at risk for social exclusion [20].

Addressing the intersection of disability and palliative care, therefore, requires a comprehensive approach that considers the unique needs of individuals with disabilities and takes an intentional approach to bridge gaps to care. This means developing new and improved ways of communicating with people with IDD and doing our best to understand and incorporate their perspectives [21]. It also means reducing social, political, cultural, and other barriers to access and communication [22]. This includes ensuring equitable access to palliative care services, providing disability-specific training for healthcare providers, and highlighting need for specialization in this area of treatment and practice [15]. By adopting an inclusive and person-centered approach, with improved strategies to minimize sensory barriers and overwhelm, and improve the likelihood of effective communication, palliative care can better meet the needs of individuals with disabilities and their families [11].

In conclusion, understanding the definition and scope of disability, the principles of palliative care, and the intersection of these two fields is essential for creating inclusive and equitable healthcare practices. By addressing the unique needs of individuals with disabilities and promoting global collaboration, we can improve the quality of life for all individuals across many diverse backgrounds [8].

2.4 Unique needs of dying individuals with disabilities

People with disabilities face unique challenges at the end of life, which require tailored approaches to care. People with intellectual and developmental disabilities (IDD) may struggle to understand aspects of their terminal condition, express their needs, and participate in decision-making processes. They may have a guardian or other decision maker who may also not reside with them. All of this can lead to significant barriers in receiving appropriate care and support [11]. Caregivers and healthcare providers must be trained to recognize and address the specific needs of individuals with IDD and also build relationships with caregivers, if one is present, to ensure their comfort and dignity during palliative care [1]. An additional barrier is that many people with IDD experience social isolation and may pass away in a group home or nursing home that specializes in serving people with IDD, which may not be located in the same community as their family, or their family may have separated themselves from their relative with a disability [23]. This means that sometimes group home staff or nursing facility staff may become like family or at least primary caregivers to some with IDD, making it important to build relationships and gain perspectives from these staff members as well.

People with physical disabilities face barriers that affect their mobility and physical functioning and ability to live independently. At the end of life, they may experience increased pain, discomfort, and challenges in accessing appropriate care. Ensuring that palliative care settings are accessible and equipped to meet their needs is crucial for providing equitable care [10]. This includes addressing mobility barriers, providing assistive devices, and individualizing care plans to accommodate physical limitations [8].

Sensory disabilities, such as vision and hearing impairments, can significantly impact an individual's end-of-life experience. There may be other types of sensory challenges outside of these conditions and these may be experienced by individuals with IDD. Sensory challenges or difficulty with touch present unique opportunities to provide a soothing environment and train on communication strategies to best understand touch options, with people with autism often preferring deep pressure touch, though each person is unique [24].

Communication barriers are a primary concern for people with sensory disabilities and with IDD as well, as both groups may have communication differences and may struggle to convey their needs and preferences, particularly when having increase in pain and physical symptoms [25]. Healthcare providers must be trained on and implement alternative communication methods, such as sign language, braille, and assistive listening devices, to ensure that individuals with sensory disabilities receive appropriate and compassionate care [11]. Creating a sensory-friendly environment can enhance their comfort and well-being during palliative care [2].

Effective communication is essential for providing high-quality palliative care to individuals with disabilities. Communication challenges can arise from cognitive impairments, speech difficulties, and sensory disabilities [1]. Healthcare providers must be skilled in using alternative communication methods, such as picture boards, communication devices, and simplified language, to facilitate meaningful interactions with patients [5]. Ensuring that individuals with disabilities can express their needs, preferences, and concerns is vital for delivering person-centered care [25].

Social differences and social isolation are additional significant challenges faced by individuals with disabilities, which can be exacerbated at the end of life. Social isolation can lead to feelings of loneliness, depression, and anxiety, negatively impacting the individual's quality of life [7]. Promoting inclusion and social support is essential for enhancing the well-being of dying individuals with disabilities. This can be achieved through community engagement, peer support programs, and involving family members and caregivers in the care process [8]. Creating an inclusive and supportive environment helps ensure that individuals with disabilities feel valued and connected during their final days [2].

Additionally, the medical model often focuses on deficits and challenges of people with disabilities. While it is important to know barriers to better inform change, it is crucial to highlight a strengths perspective that embraces the strengths and individuality of each person with a disability [22]. Elevating the voices of people with IDD wherever possible helps to better see and understand their unique strengths. For example, a nonspeaking individual may be assumed to have an intellectual disability, but evidence shows they may have strong thinking and reasoning skills and can communicate via keyboard [26]. Not making assumptions and getting to know the unique individual they are serving, and the best ways to approach and communicate, makes a huge difference in building trust and providing quality care [27].

Addressing the unique needs of dying individuals with disabilities requires a comprehensive and compassionate approach. By recognizing and addressing the specific challenges faced by individuals with IDD, physical disabilities, and sensory disabilities, healthcare providers can deliver equitable and person-centered palliative care. Effective communication and promoting inclusion are key components of providing high-quality end-of-life care for individuals with disabilities [11]. Through these efforts, we can improve the quality of life for all individuals, regardless of their abilities or backgrounds [8].

2.5 Marginalization and intersectionality

Marginalization and intersectionality are critical concepts in understanding the unique challenges faced by individuals with disabilities, particularly at the end of life. Marginalization occurs when individuals or groups are pushed to the edges of society, limiting their access to resources, opportunities, and rights [28]. This is often compounded by factors such as race, culture, and socioeconomic status, which intersect to create complex layers of disadvantage [5]. For example, individuals from minority ethnic backgrounds or lower socioeconomic statuses may face additional barriers to accessing palliative care, resulting in poorer health outcomes and reduced quality of life [8]. Additionally, they are less likely to be able to afford caregivers, meaning that they have higher likelihood of needing to go to a nursing facility even if their wish was to pass away in the comfort of their home surrounded by loved ones [29].

The concept of intersectionality, introduced by Kimberlé Crenshaw in 1989, provides a framework for understanding how multiple forms of discrimination and oppression overlap and intersect [4]. Intersectionality highlights that individuals do not experience discrimination in isolation; rather, their experiences are shaped by the interplay of various social identities, such as race, gender, disability, and socioeconomic status [4]. This framework is particularly relevant in palliative care, where the compounded effects of multiple marginalizations can significantly impact the care and support individuals receive and that we must also pay attention to how multiple aspects of marginalization may uniquely impact someone [5].

Applying a critical disability justice lens further deepens our understanding of these issues. Critical disability studies challenge traditional views of disability, emphasizing the social and political dimensions of disability rather than merely focusing on medical or individual impairments [30]. This perspective calls for a shift from viewing disability as a deficit to recognizing it as a dimension of human diversity that intersects with other social identities [31]. By adopting this lens, we can better address the systemic inequities and power imbalances that contribute to the marginalization of individuals with disabilities [32].

In the context of palliative care, these frameworks underscore the importance of addressing the unique needs of individuals with disabilities through inclusive and equitable practices. For instance, healthcare providers must be aware of the cultural and socioeconomic factors that influence access to care and work to eliminate barriers that prevent marginalized groups from receiving appropriate support [1]. This includes providing culturally competent care, ensuring accessibility, and advocating for policies that promote health equity [7].

Moreover, intersectionality and critical disability justice highlight the need for collaborative efforts to address these challenges. By engaging with diverse communities and incorporating their perspectives into palliative care practices, we can create more inclusive and responsive care systems [5]. This approach not only improves the quality of care for individuals with disabilities but also fosters a more just and equitable society [8].

Understanding marginalization and intersectionality is essential for addressing the unique challenges faced by individuals with disabilities in palliative care. By applying the intersectionality framework and a critical disability justice lens, we can better recognize and address the compounded injustices experienced by marginalized individuals. This approach calls for inclusive and equitable practices that consider the diverse needs of individuals with disabilities, ultimately improving their quality of life and ensuring that they receive the care and support they deserve [5].

3. Disparities in palliative care

Disparities in palliative care significantly affect various racial and cultural groups. Individuals from minority ethnic backgrounds often face systemic barriers that limit their access to quality healthcare. These barriers include socioeconomic factors, geographic location, and a lack of culturally competent care providers [5]. Cultural beliefs and practices also play a crucial role in how different communities perceive and engage with palliative care services. For instance, some cultures may prioritize family involvement in care decisions, while others may have specific rituals and practices related to end-of-life care [8]. Understanding and respecting these cultural differences is essential for providing effective and compassionate palliative care.

Black/African American individuals, in particular, have historically faced and continue to face numerous barriers to accessing quality palliative care. These barriers are often compounded by systemic racism and socioeconomic disadvantages. Historically, Black Americans have been subjected to discriminatory practices that have excluded them from receiving adequate healthcare, and these injustices have left a lasting impact on their health outcomes [33]. For example, the harm and trauma of the Tuskegee Syphilis Study contributed greatly to a mistrust of the healthcare system among Black communities, which can deter individuals from seeking palliative care [34].

Access to care is a fundamental aspect of palliative care, yet Black individuals often encounter systemic obstacles that limit their access. These barriers include socioeconomic factors, geographic location, and a lack of culturally competent care providers [34]. Studies have shown that Black patients are less likely to receive hospice care and more likely to undergo aggressive treatments at the end of life compared to their White counterparts [35]. This disparity in care quality can be attributed to a lack of trust in the healthcare system, stemming from historical abuses and ongoing experiences of discrimination and bias in medical settings [34]. These factors contribute to a reluctance among Black individuals to engage with palliative care services, resulting in poorer health outcomes and increased suffering [36].

Quality of care is another critical area where disparities are evident. Black patients often receive lower quality care compared to their White counterparts, which can result in inadequate pain management, lack of emotional support, and insufficient communication about care options [35]. These disparities in care quality can exacerbate the suffering of Black patients and their families during the end-of-life process [36].

Cultural competence and humility in healthcare is essential for addressing these disparities. Cultural competence and cultural humility involve understanding and respecting cultural differences and needs of patients and an open curiosity of learning from patients of diverse backgrounds, which is crucial for providing effective palliative care [5]. However, many healthcare providers lack the training and awareness needed to deliver culturally competent care, leading to misunderstandings and inadequate support for Black patients [8]. For example, Black families may prioritize life-prolonging interventions due to cultural and religious beliefs, yet healthcare providers may not fully understand or respect these preferences, resulting in conflicts and suboptimal care [36].

The intersection of race, culture, and socioeconomic status further compounds these disparities. Black individuals are more likely to live in poverty and have limited access to healthcare resources, which exacerbates their challenges in receiving palliative care [37]. Additionally, systemic racism and implicit biases within the healthcare system continue to affect the quality of care that Black patients receive, often in more covert ways than in the past [34]. These ongoing injustices highlight the need for comprehensive efforts to address the root causes of disparities in palliative care and to promote equity and inclusion in healthcare [33].

Disability and older adulthood add additional layers of marginalization. Evidence shows that people with IDD and seniors have higher rates of trauma, abuse, bullying, social exclusion, and untreated pain due to communication challenges or stigma [38].

4. Global perspectives

Understanding global perspectives on disability and palliative care is crucial for developing inclusive and equitable practices that address the diverse needs of individuals worldwide [5]. Different regions and cultures have unique approaches to palliative care, influenced by their healthcare systems, cultural beliefs, and socioeconomic conditions. By examining case studies from various regions, though these examples do not show the rich cultural diversity worldwide nor the deep diversity within diverse populations, we can gain insights into the challenges and successes of different palliative care practices and identify opportunities for global collaboration and improvement [5].

4.1 Case example 1: Palliative care for individuals with disabilities in India

In India, palliative care services are still developing, and access to care is limited, particularly for individuals with disabilities. A case study of a young woman with cerebral palsy highlights the challenges faced by individuals with disabilities in accessing palliative care. Despite her significant physical limitations, she lived in a rural area with limited healthcare infrastructure. Her family struggled to find appropriate care and support, and cultural stigmas surrounding disability further compounded their difficulties [39]. Through the efforts of a local non-governmental organization (NGO), the family received home-based palliative care, which included pain management, physical therapy, and emotional support. This case highlights the importance of community-based initiatives and the need for culturally sensitive care that addresses the unique needs of individuals with disabilities in low-resource settings [39].

4.2 Case example 2: Palliative care for individuals with disabilities in Sweden

Sweden has a comprehensive healthcare system and strong social support networks [40]. A case study of an elderly man with intellectual and developmental disabilities (IDD) receiving palliative care in Sweden illustrates the benefits of an inclusive and well-resourced healthcare system. The man lived in a group home with access to specialized healthcare providers trained in both palliative care and disability support. His care plan was developed collaboratively with input from his family, caregivers, and healthcare team, ensuring that his physical, emotional, and social needs were met [40]. This case highlights the importance of interdisciplinary collaboration and the positive impact of a supportive healthcare infrastructure on the quality of palliative care for individuals with disabilities [40].

4.3 Comparative analysis of palliative care practices

Comparing palliative care practices across different regions reveals significant disparities in access, quality, and cultural competence. In high-income countries like Sweden, individuals with disabilities often benefit from well-established healthcare systems and comprehensive support services. In contrast, low- and middle-income countries like India face challenges related to limited resources, inadequate healthcare infrastructure, and cultural stigmas [39, 40]. These disparities highlight the need for global efforts to better understand and improve palliative care access and quality, particularly for marginalized populations [5].

4.4 Global contributions and collaborations

Global contributions and collaborations are essential for addressing the disparities in palliative care for individuals with disabilities [41]. International organizations, such as the World Health Organization (WHO), play a crucial role in promoting best practices, providing technical assistance, and supporting capacity-building initiatives in low-resource settings [41]. Collaborative efforts between countries can facilitate the exchange of knowledge, resources, and expertise, leading to improved palliative care practices worldwide [8]. For example, partnerships between NGOs in India and healthcare institutions in high-income countries have led to the development of innovative community-based palliative care models that address the unique needs of individuals with disabilities [39].

4.5 Questions for reflection

1. How do cultural beliefs and practices influence the provision of palliative care for individuals with disabilities in different regions?

2. What are the key challenges faced by individuals with disabilities in accessing palliative care in low- and middle-income countries?

3. How can interdisciplinary collaboration improve the quality of palliative care for individuals with disabilities?

4. What role do international organizations and global collaborations play in addressing disparities in palliative care?

5. How can healthcare providers ensure that palliative care practices are culturally sensitive and inclusive? How do we learn to practice cultural humility?

By considering these questions, we reflect on the complexities of providing palliative care for individuals with disabilities and the importance of a global perspective in addressing these challenges.

4.6 Advocacy and policy recommendations

Advocacy and policy recommendations are essential for creating inclusive palliative care practices that address the diverse needs of individuals with disabilities. Strategies for inclusive palliative care involve ensuring equitable access to services, enhancing the quality of care, and fostering cultural competence among healthcare providers. One effective strategy is to implement community-based palliative care models that provide care in patients' homes and communities, making services more accessible to individuals with disabilities [39]. Additionally, training healthcare providers in disability-specific needs and cultural competence can improve the quality of care and ensure that patients receive respectful and appropriate support [5].

Policy changes at both the national and global levels are crucial for advancing inclusive palliative care. In the United States, the Palliative Care and Hospice Education and Training Act (PCHETA) aims to expand the palliative care workforce, increase research funding, and raise public awareness about palliative care [42]. This legislation is essential for addressing workforce shortages and improving the quality of palliative care services. At the state level, policymakers can support initiatives such as loan forgiveness programs for palliative care specialists and grants for remote consultations in rural areas, which can help address disparities in access to care [42].

Globally, international organizations like the World Health Organization (WHO) and the Worldwide Hospice Palliative Care Alliance (WHPCA) play a vital role in promoting best practices and supporting capacity-building initiatives in low-resource settings [41]. Collaborative efforts between countries can facilitate the exchange of knowledge, resources, and expertise, leading to improved palliative care practices worldwide [8]. For example, partnerships between non-governmental organizations (NGOs) in low- and middle-income countries and healthcare institutions in high-income countries have led to the development of innovative community-based palliative care models that address the unique needs of individuals with disabilities [39].

Social workers and caregivers play a critical role in providing palliative care for individuals with disabilities and from various marginalized backgrounds. Social workers address the social, emotional, and psychological needs of patients and their families, helping them navigate the complexities of end-of-life care [43]. They provide counseling, facilitate advance care planning, and advocate for patients' rights and preferences [43]. Social workers provide care in areas of end of life care and disability, to name a few [43]. Caregivers, including family members and professional caregivers, offer essential support in managing daily activities, providing emotional comfort, and ensuring that patients' needs are met [44]. By working collaboratively with healthcare providers, social workers and caregivers can enhance the quality of palliative care and ensure that individuals with disabilities receive culturally sensitive, inclusive, comprehensive and compassionate support [45].

5. Conclusion

In summary, this chapter explores the intersection of disability and palliative care from a global perspective, highlighting the unique needs of dying individuals with disabilities and the compounded injustices they face. By examining the concepts of marginalization and intersectionality, we underscore the importance of addressing the diverse needs of individuals with disabilities through inclusive and equitable palliative care practices [5]. The case studies from different regions have illustrates the challenges and successes of various palliative care practices, emphasizing the need for global collaboration and knowledge exchange [39, 40].

A call to action for global collaboration and change is essential for improving palliative care for individuals with disabilities. International organizations, governments, and healthcare providers must work together to promote best practices, support capacity-building initiatives, and advocate for policy changes that enhance access to quality palliative care [41]. By fostering interdisciplinary collaboration and engaging with diverse communities, we can create more inclusive and responsive care systems that address the unique needs of individuals with disabilities [8].

Future directions for research and practice in palliative care should focus on addressing the gaps in knowledge and improving the quality of care for individuals with disabilities. This includes conducting rigorous clinical trials to build the evidence base for palliative care interventions, exploring innovative care models, and developing culturally competent care practices [46]. Additionally, research should examine the impact of social determinants of health on palliative care outcomes and identify strategies to address these factors [47]. By advancing research and practice in these areas, and grounding our work in the voices of people with disabilities, we strive for social justice, inclusion, and the compassionate and comprehensive care persons with disabilities deserve at end of life [48].

Resources

Palliative Care and Intellectual Disabilities | Intellectual Disability and Health: This resource provides comprehensive information on palliative care for individuals with intellectual disabilities, including pain management, communication, and end-of-life decision-making.

Supporting Families of People With IDD: A National Community of Practice: This resource offers tools and guidance for developing and improving support systems for families of individuals with IDD, including policy recommendations and practical strategies.

Intellectual and Developmental Disabilities (IDDs) Resources | NICHD - Eunice Kennedy Shriver National Institute of Child Health and Human Development: This page provides links to various organizations and resources that offer information and support for individuals with IDD and their families, including end-of-life care.

Bereavement—A guide for autistic adults: The National Autistic Society offers a guide to help autistic adults cope with bereavement, including practical tips and support strategies.

Grief and Loss Resources | Autism Alliance: Autism Alliance provides grief and loss resources and community supports for loved ones with autism, including a list of certified Autism Welcoming™ funeral homes.

Thank you

Sincere thank you to all I have learned from mentors and colleagues but, most importantly, from people with intellectual and developmental disability including my Aunt Karen and my son Tommy. I am better for your contributions and your love.

Author details

Jessica Curd
Indiana University, Indianapolis, United States

*Address all correspondence to: jschoett@iu.edu

References

[1] Koffman J, Shapiro GK, Schulz-Quach C. Enhancing equity and diversity in palliative care clinical practice, research, and education. BMC Palliative Care. 2023;**22**(64)

[2] Jansen-van Vuuren J, Aldersey HM. Stigma, acceptance, and belonging for people with IDD across cultures. Current Developmental Disorders Reports. 2020;**7**(3):163-172

[3] Ghoshal A, Damani A. Palliative care for people with physical and intellectual disabilities. The Palgrave Encyclopedia of Disability. 2025

[4] Crenshaw K. On Intersectionality: Essential Writings. New York, NY: The New Press; 2017

[5] Butler H, Gott M, Prebble K, Fortune S, Robinson J. Palliative care research utilising intersectionality: A scoping review. BMC Palliative Care. 2023;**22**:189

[6] Presnell J, Keesler J, Curd J, Carroll D. Promoting justice for people with intellectual and developmental disabilities: Strategies for advancing anti-oppressive social work education and practice. Journal of Sociology and Social Welfare. 2024;**51**(1):Article 8. Available from: https://scholarworks.wmich.edu/jssw/vol51/iss1/8

[7] Peeler A, Afolabi O, Harding R. Palliative care is an overlooked global health priority. BMJ. 2024;**387**:q2387

[8] Walker ME. Global perspectives: Palliative care around the world. In: Holtslander L, Peacock S, Bally J, editors. Hospice Palliative Home Care and Bereavement Support. Cham: Springer; 2019. pp. 121-136

[9] World Health Organization (WHO). World Report on Disability. 2011. Available from: https://www.who.int/disabilities/world_report/2011/report.pdf

[10] Centers for Disease Control and Prevention (CDC). Disability and Health Overview. 2024. Available from: https://www.cdc.gov/ncbddd/disabilityandhealth/index.html

[11] Dong MY, Meredith L, Forrester-Jones R, Kothari A, Ryan D, Ryan BL, et al. Individualized participatory care planning for individuals with intellectual and developmental disabilities: A qualitative descriptive study. BMC Health Services Research. 2024;**24**

[12] Masel EK, Antunes B, Schulz-Quach C. Palliative care in severe mental illnesses. BMC Palliative Care. 2023;**22**:Article 31

[13] Cleveland Clinic. Palliative Care: Overview and Benefits. 2024. Available from: https://my.clevelandclinic.org/health/treatments/21076-palliative-care

[14] National Institute on Aging. Palliative Care: Improving Quality of Life for Patients and Families. 2024. Available from: https://www.nia.nih.gov/health/palliative-care

[15] Sítima G, Galhardo-Branco C, Reis-Pina P. Equity of access to palliative care: A scoping review. International Journal for Equity in Health. 2024;**23**:248. Available from: https://equityhealthj.biomedcentral.com/articles/10.1186/s12939-024-02321-1

[16] Mayo Clinic. End-of-Life Care. 2023. Available from: https://www.mayoclinic.org/healthy-lifestyle/end-of-life/basics/endoflife-care/hlv-20049403

[17] National Hospice and Palliative Care Organization (NHPCO). Palliative Care: Multidisciplinary Team Approach. 2023. Available from: https://www.nhpco.org/palliative-care/

[18] Stanford Medicine. Palliative Care: A Multidisciplinary Approach. 2021. Available from: https://med.stanford.edu/palliative-care.html

[19] Adam E, Sleeman KE, Brearley S, Hunt K, Tuffrey-Wijne I. The palliative care needs of adults with intellectual disabilities and their access to palliative care services: A systematic review. Palliative Medicine. 2020;**34**(8):1006-1018

[20] Taylor HO, Cudjoe TKM, Bu F, Lim MH. The state of loneliness and social isolation research: Current knowledge and future directions. BMC Public Health. 2023;**23**:1049. Available from: https://bmcpublichealth.biomedcentral.com/articles/10.1186/s12889-023-15967-3

[21] Sue K, Mazzotta P, Grier E. Palliative care for patients with communication and cognitive difficulties. Canadian Family Physician. 2019;**65**(Suppl 1):S19-S23

[22] Engel M, Kars MC, Teunissen SCCM, van der Heide A. Effective communication in palliative care from the perspectives of patients and relatives: A systematic review. Palliative & Supportive Care. 2023;**21**(5):890-913

[23] Covey H. Loneliness: What It Means for Individuals with Disabilities. Covey Insights; 2020

[24] Backman C, Demery-Varin M, Cho-Young D, Crick M, Squires J. Impact of sensory interventions on the quality of life of long-term care residents: A scoping review. BMJ Open. 2021;**11**(3):e042466

[25] Disability Support Guide. Sensory Disabilities: Challenges and Solutions. Disability Support Guide; 2023. Available from: https://www.disabilitysupportguide.com.au/information/article/sensory-disabilities

[26] Terao T, Satoh M. The present state of existential interventions within palliative care. Frontiers in Psychiatry. 2021;**12**:Article 811612

[27] Ekberg S, Parry R, Land V, Ekberg K, Pino M, Antaki C, et al. Communicating with patients and families about illness progression and end of life: A review of studies using direct observation of clinical practice. BMC Palliative Care. 2021;**20**:Article 186

[28] Wolbring G, Nasir L. Intersectionality of disabled people through a disability studies, ability-based studies, and intersectional pedagogy lens: A survey and a scoping review. Societies. 2024;**14**(9):Article 176

[29] Aker N, Griffiths S, Kupeli N, Frost R, Nair P, Walters K, et al. Experiences and access of palliative and end of life care for older people from minority ethnic groups: A scoping review. BMC Palliative Care. 2024;**23**:Article 228

[30] Robinson S. Moving toward disability justice. Disability Studies Quarterly. 2017;**32**(3)

[31] Flynn S. Critical disability studies. In: The Palgrave Encyclopedia of Disability. Springer; 2024. pp. 1-6

[32] Gréaux M, Moro MF, Kamenov K, Russell AM, Barrett D, Cieza A. Health equity for persons with disabilities: A global scoping review on barriers and interventions in healthcare services. International Journal for Equity in Health. 2023;**22**:Article 236

[33] Smithsonian Institution. The Legacy of the Tuskegee Syphilis Study and Its Impact on Black Americans' Trust in Healthcare. 2022. Available from: https://www.si.edu

[34] Kaiser Family Foundation (KFF). Barriers to Palliative Care for Black Americans. 2024. Available from: https://www.kff.org

[35] Johns Hopkins Medicine. Disparities in End-of-Life Care for Black Patients. 2020. Available from: https://www.hopkinsmedicine.org

[36] Association of American Medical Colleges (AAMC). Addressing Disparities in Palliative Care for Black Patients. 2022. Available from: https://www.aamc.org

[37] Healthline. The Impact of Socioeconomic Status on Palliative Care Access. 2024. Available from: https://www.healthline.com

[38] Harvey K. Trauma-informed care for people with intellectual disabilities. In: End Abuse of People with Disabilities. 2021

[39] Rathore P, Kumar S, Gupta R. Palliative care practices in India: Challenges and opportunities. Indian Journal of Palliative Care. 2024

[40] Ågren A, Krevers B, Cedersund E, Nedlund A-C. Policy narratives on palliative care in Sweden 1974-2018. Health Care Analysis. 2023;**31**(1):99-113

[41] World Health Organization (WHO). Promoting Best Practices in Palliative Care. 2022. Available from: https://www.who.int

[42] Center to Advance Palliative Care (CAPC). Palliative Care and Hospice Education and Training Act (PCHETA). 2024. Available from: https://www.capc.org

[43] National Association of Social Workers (NASW). Standards for Palliative and End of Life Care. 2024. Available from: https://www.socialworkers.org/Practice/NASW-Practice-Standards-Guidelines/Standards-for-Palliative-and-End-of-Life-Care

[44] Engrace Hospice. The Role of Caregivers in Palliative Care. 2024. Available from: https://www.engracehospice.com

[45] Pornrattanakavee P, Srichan T, Seetalarom K, Saichaemchan S, Oer-areemitr N, Prasongsook N. Impact of interprofessional collaborative practice in palliative care on outcomes for advanced cancer inpatients in a resource-limited setting. BMC Palliative Care. 2022;**21**:Article 229

[46] Patient-Centered Outcomes Research Institute (PCORI). Building the Evidence Base for Palliative Care Interventions. 2024. Available from: https://www.pcori.org

[47] National Institute of Nursing Research (NINR). Social Determinants of Health and Palliative Care Outcomes. 2024. Available from: https://www.ninr.nih.gov

[48] Pfaff K, Markaki A. Compassionate collaborative care: An integrative review of quality indicators in end-of-life care. BMC Palliative Care. 2017;**16**:Article 65

Chapter 2

Perspective Chapter: The Healing Bond – Using Interdisciplinary Teams to Increase Emotional Intelligence and Improve Serious Illness Care

Terrance Ruth

Abstract

Serious illness care as a field of practice could benefit from teaching and learning about emotional intelligence as a means for advancing the healing bond and other holistic intervention. Holistic therapies empower the patient and family to actively engage in their own care with in ways that help them to feel seen and hear in the caring process. Arguably, the evolving landscape of hospice and palliative care necessitates a balanced amalgamation of technical proficiency and emotional intelligence (EI). Emotional intelligence, defined as the ability to identify, comprehend, and manage one's own emotions and those of others, is pivotal in the healthcare context. It enhances patient-provider relationships, leading to improved care quality and patient satisfaction. This chapter will examine the role of EI in serious illness care, particularly how an interdisciplinary can enhance EI awareness through social work leadership, thereby improving patient outcomes. The focus areas include understanding patient needs, reducing patient anxiety, and advocating for patients. Three research questions are explored in order to shed light on the role of EI in serious illness care, emphasizing the importance of collaboration between healthcare professionals and social workers in fostering emotional intelligence and, ultimately, improving patient outcomes. Lastly, the chapter concludes with finding and recommendations for culturally competent practices for an interdisciplinary field of practitioners in serious illness care.

Keywords: emotional intelligence, communication, patient advocacy, cultural awareness, cultural competency

1. Introduction

In order to meet the needs and care demand of a culturally diverse patient population, interdisciplinary health care teams may benefit from incorporating emotional intelligence (EI) as a crucial skill that enables them to comprehend and effectively manage their own emotions as well as those of their patients when caring for seriously ill patients who also may be at end of life [1]. Research that examines the association between EI in healthcare settings and explores how collaborations among the interprofessional team can be strengthened warrants attention through a lens of innovative operationalization and practice frameworks. Emotional intelligence is suggested as a tool that can be used in the formation of professional-patient relationship, resulting in better care quality and patient satisfaction. By developing EI skills, healthcare professionals may increase their understanding of culturally-bounded patient needs, reduce patient anxiety, and facilitate essential advocacy on behalf of the patient and family [1, 2]. Thus, the research study discussed in this chapter aims to shed light on the role of EI in healthcare, emphasizing the importance of collaboration between serious illness care professionals with a particular emphasizes on the role of social workers leading with emotional intelligence and, ultimately, improving patient outcomes.

2. Background

The evolving landscape of healthcare necessitates a balanced amalgamation of technical proficiency and emotional intelligence (EI). Emotional intelligence, defined as the ability to identify, comprehend, and manage one's own emotions and those of others, is pivotal in the healthcare context. It enhances patient-provider relationships, leading to improved care quality and patient satisfaction. This chapter discusses the role of EI in healthcare, particularly how social workers can enhance EI awareness among healthcare professionals, thereby improving patient outcomes. The research spans a decade of evidence-based practices that support the translation of the work to serious illness care that center social work practitioners [3, 4]. Moreover, the emphasis is on basic skills of understanding patient needs, reducing patient anxiety, and advocating for patients. It fills a gap in the literature by focusing on the micro, mezzo and macro levels of interventions that may improve the quality of care that patients and families receive.

2.1 Understanding patient needs

Understanding patient needs is fundamental to providing patient-centered care. Healthcare professionals with high EI can better perceive and address the emotional and psychological needs of patients, leading to more effective and compassionate care. Research links levels of empathy and Patient Care. A study published in in the field of Psychology explores how empathy, a core component of EI, influences patient care [5]. The findings suggest that nurses with higher levels of empathy, facilitated by their emotional intelligence, are better equipped to understand and respond to patient needs, leading to higher patient satisfaction and improved health outcomes [5].

Additionally, research offers a potential understanding about health outcomes and emotional intelligence in nursing. In a different study focused emotional intelligence, self-efficacy and empathy as predictors of overall self-esteem in nursing experiences, it was revealed that nurses with higher EI are more confident in their abilities to meet patient needs and provide high-quality care [5]. The EI of clinicians impacts patient relationships and health outcomes for the patient and family. Among health care managers, a stronger EI could increase the likelihood that the clinician will be able to build strong relationships with their patients. Such strong relationships are characterized by better communication, greater trust, and a deeper understanding of patient needs, ultimately enhancing patient satisfaction and care quality [6]. Furthermore, it was argued that a part of enhancing satisfaction in serious illness care is the capacity to reduce patient anxiety. EI may have a role to play in doing so when anxiety is not left out of the treatment team equation and consider to be a common emotion experienced by patients in healthcare settings. Evidence shows that healthcare professionals with higher EI are able to recognize and alleviate patient anxiety than those with lower EI, creating a more comforting and supportive environment [6] when then may be addressed earlier in the disease course and treatment plan.

2.2 Reducing patient anxiety

In primary care we have long known that empath has a role in reducing anxiety and to integrate such knowledge and application in serious illness care can be helpful in the family meeting, education and counseling session. With EI, healthcare providers who demonstrate empathy may be able to significantly reduce patient anxiety among patients. By acknowledging and addressing patients' fears and concerns, emotionally intelligent providers create a more reassuring and less stressful healthcare experience [7]. Scholars have identified such the need for healthcare professional to draw upon their EI to developing communication plans and intervention with patient that are also experiencing anxiety. A study with a global focus highlights how effective communication, a key aspect of EI, can reduce patient anxiety, stress, cognitive load and performance. In a randomized controlled trial, dyad learning that investigated relationship between these factors concluded that such interventions are effective. Moreover, educating and training healthcare professionals in EI improves their ability to communicate clearly and empathetically, thereby reducing patient stress and improving overall satisfaction [8]. The goal of patient-centered care should be to emphasis the importance of and incorporate emotional support [9] and in serious illness care such as hospice, palliative and end-of-life care it is all the more important [10]. Engaging in the clinical work that that explores mid-level, community interventions, and macro level policies may be essential to bring about long-term change. Noteworthy is the fact that the importance of emotional support in healthcare has not always been effectively incorporated into the training of healthcare teams. Yet, this research suggests that healthcare professionals who provide emotional support, facilitated by their EI, can help mitigate patient anxiety and promote a more positive healthcare experience as has previous research [11].

2.3 Advocating for patients

Advocacy is another important aspect of serious illness care, ensuring that patients' needs and preferences are respected and met. Healthcare professionals with high EI are better advocates, as they can understand and articulate patients' concerns and preferences more effectively. Advocacy and Emotional Intelligence are interconnected. According to a study in Nursing Ethics, clinicians with high EI are more effective advocates for their patients [2, 12, 13]. They can navigate complex emotional and ethical situations, ensuring that patients' voices are heard and their rights are protected [12]. The focus on patient-centered care and advocacy narrows the concentration on professional-client relationship. Research published in the Journal of Advanced Nursing emphasizes the role of EI in patient-centered care [14]. Healthcare professionals with high EI are more attuned to their patients' needs and preferences, enabling them to advocate more effectively for their patients and improve care outcomes [14].

Social Workers, in particular, are likely to be in the position of advocating for patients and families faced with serious illness care. Such advocacy can influence the type of relationship that the clinician develops the patient and the specific outcomes. Evidence-based practices are essential. In research focused on innovations in efficient, effective and quality oriented practices and procedures with social workers, it was argued that creative strategies that streamlined, well-organized and efficeint practices that are quality driven and multi-dimensional are needed [15]. It is believed that clinicians trained in EI will be ideally suited as interprofessional team members in serious illness care to enhance patient care and champion this innovation, especially with culturally diverse populations [16]. As members of interdisciplinary teams, social workers and other serious illness care providers can ensure that patients receive comprehensive and compassionate care that respects their individual needs and preferences [15]. This will likely require going beyond the standard of cultural humility to extend the awareness, skills and transferrable knowledge needed to develop patient-centered, culturally concordant care plans [17] that is guided by innovative tools that are designed to close gaps in patients' access to care [18]. The integration of emotional intelligence into hospice, palliative and end-of-life care practices may advance the field towards addressing barriers that have long existed in the field and perpetuated disparities in care outcomes to create greater representation [19] and culturally competent practitioners [17] which are crucial for enhancing patient care and outcomes. Social workers play a vital role in fostering EI awareness among healthcare professionals [1]. By improving EI skills, clinicians can better understand patient needs, reduce patient anxiety, and advocate effectively for their patients. Centering EI is a collaborative approach that not only improves the quality of care but also ensures a more compassionate and patient-centered healthcare environment [20].

2.4 The facts

The integration of Emotional Intelligence (EI) in healthcare practice has gained significant attention due to its profound impact on patient outcomes and healthcare provider well-being [21]. For decades, there is evidence that suggests emotional intelligence is associated with a range of positive outcomes, the ability to provide compassionate and competent care for patients and families, as well as to provide essential leadership [22] the ability to lead and influence others, and the ability to manage stress, all of which are important in pharmacy education. This analysis examines the assumptions and proposed strategies for social workers and health professionals. By delving into the assumptions, the role of social workers is emphasized because of their education and training which centers social justice approaches to care [20, 23], and the suggested strategies that elucidate the potential benefits and challenges of incorporating EI as a necessary component of care for patients with serious illness in hospice, palliative and end-of-life care.

3. Research questions addressed by evidence in the literature

The first questions in about whether or not an increase in EI in interprofessional care clinicians will lead to greater patient satisfaction. The scholarship posits that higher EI in medical professionals enhances patient satisfaction. This first assumption is supported by multiple studies indicating that emotionally intelligent healthcare providers can better understand and meet patient needs. For instance, physicians and nurses with high EI are more empathetic, leading to more meaningful interactions with patients [24]. This empathetic approach fosters trust and a deeper connection, which are crucial for patient satisfaction [25]. Moreover, when healthcare providers exhibit high EI, they can tailor their communication to be more patient-centered, ensuring that patients feel heard and valued. This personalized care approach is likely to result in higher patient satisfaction [26].

The second questions is about whether or not the increase in emotional intelligence (EI) among interprofessional clinicians will lead to higher interpersonal relationships. Interpersonal relationships within healthcare teams are vital for effective patient care. The assumption that increased EI among medical professionals leads to improved interpersonal relationships is well-founded. High EI enables healthcare providers to navigate complex emotional and social dynamics, promoting better teamwork and collaboration [26]. For example, emotionally intelligent professionals are more adept at managing conflicts and understanding the perspectives of their colleagues [27]. This skill is crucial in a healthcare setting where multidisciplinary collaboration is necessary for comprehensive patient care. Additionally, strong interpersonal relationships within healthcare teams can enhance job satisfaction and reduce burnout, further improving the quality of care provided [27].

The third questions is about whether or not an increase in emotional intelligence (EI) among interprofessional clinicians will lead to improved stress management. Research scholars have documented the benefit of EI in medical education including pharmacy training [21]. They argue that greater EI in medical professionals, the more likely it is that they will be able to manage stress. This assumption is supported by research indicating that EI equips individuals with the tools to recognize and regulate their own emotions effectively [24]. Most serious illness clinicians would argue that they work in high-stress environments. Thus, the work of Wiechula et al. [14] is particularly relevant for serious illness clinicians. It suggests that EI offers professionals a key ingredient for managing stress, which is related to one's capacity to accurately appraise and express emotions in oneself and in others, and then, to effectively regulate those emotions by using feelings to motivate, guide and act in ways that are calming and non-disruptive to self and others [22]. EI allows one to maintain composure, patience, and resilience in the face of challenging situations. Furthermore, emotionally intelligent clinicians are better equipped to support their colleagues, creating a more supportive and less stressful work environment [14]. This improved stress management can lead to reduced burnout and improved overall well-being for healthcare professionals [14].

This research proposes three potential benefits to leveraging social workers, specifically, in leading the charge of enhancing EI awareness among healthcare professionals [1]. The first benefit includes social workers trained in emotional intelligence and the influence they have on other health professionals. Social workers are uniquely educated and prepared to lead EI initiatives in healthcare settings due to their training and ethical commitments [3, 23, 28]. Social work education emphasizes empathy, ethical decision-making, and emotional regulation, making social workers well-suited to model and teach EI skills. By integrating EI training into social work practice, social workers can lead by example and demonstrate the benefits of high EI in patient care and team dynamics [29]. This approach aligns with the ethical standards of the social work profession, which emphasize respect for individuals' dignity and the importance of human relationships [16].

The second benefit includes social workers as trainers and advisers to hospice, palliative and end-of-life care in emotional intelligence. Social workers can play a pivotal role in training and advising palliative care teams [10, 30]. Through workshops, seminars, and one-on-one coaching, social workers can impart essential EI skills to healthcare providers. This training can include techniques for recognizing and managing emotions, improving communication, and building empathy. Additionally, social workers can provide ongoing support and mentorship to medical professionals, helping them apply EI principles in their daily practice. This continuous professional development ensures that healthcare providers remain proficient in EI skills and can adapt to the evolving needs of their patients [29].

The third benefit includes social workers as skilled clinicians to address and support the intersectionality of racial, ethnic, social, and other differences in hospice, palliative and end-of-life (EOL) care. This is imperative in ethical serious illness care given the ever growing range of diversity characteristics among the increasing populations of culturally diverse individuals and families, globally that face stress when living with serious illness. Supporting stress management is among the most important roles of social workers and is critical contribution to palliative care teams and patients [16]. When social workers offer counseling services to seriously ill patients, stress management a part of the services provided, which can be facilitate through stress management workshops, and peer support groups, and other strategies for mitigating high levels of stress and may extend to our colleagues who may be experiencing burnout in serious illness care. They need support in order to maintain resilience to sustain their capacity to provide care for patients who may need it the most, patients with incurable illness [3, 29]. These interventions not only support individual healthcare providers but also contribute to a healthier and more resilient workforce. When health care providers are better equipped to manage their stress, they can provide higher quality care to their patients and work more effectively with their colleagues [31] and social workers, as health care clinicians have an ethical obligation to develop and sustain specialized knowledge and understanding about history, traditions, values and family systems as these are essential components to effective palliative and end-of-life care outcomes [32].

The integration of emotional intelligence into hospice, palliative and end-of-life care, facilitated by social workers, holds significant promise for improving patient care and healthcare provider well-being. The assumptions that higher levels of EI will lead to increased patient satisfaction, better interpersonal relationships, and improved stress management are well-supported by existing research [33]. Social workers, with their preparation to be empathic and ethical practice, are ideally positioned to lead EI initiatives in healthcare settings. By training and advising interdisciplinary professionals in EI and supporting stress management efforts, social workers can help create a more emotionally intelligent contexts for patient care and effective health outcomes. This collaborative approach not only enhances the quality of patient care but also fosters a more supportive and sustainable work environment for interprofessional clinicians in hospice, palliative and serious illness care for patients and families that have been historically marginalized in palliative care research and practice [19].

4. Discussion and future direction for cultural competence in palliative care

As hospice, palliative and end of life care continues to be a growing field of practice, and social workers continue to center social justice, health equity and patient-center practices, the need for culturally competent clinician will remain. Thus, as palliative care clinicians continue to grapple with the gaps in care for culturally diverse patient population, the challenge is to understand what is necessary in order to provide equitable care to diverse populations of patients and their families. This will mean that specialized palliative care clinicians must be attentive to meet the needs of person living with life-limiting illness that tend to underutilize hospice, palliative and end-of-life and bereavement care [17]. Emotional intelligence (EI) has been shown to be worthwhile in helping clinicians to close some of the gaps in what has been considered to culturally incongruent care. Care paradigms that support teaching and educating clinicians about differences in patients' preferences for and against care will improve patient outcomes [1, 16]. Furthermore, EI can support clinicians in dealing with the inevitable moral distress that emerges in hospice, palliative and end-of-life care for persons that may need the greatest level of attention and compassion, especially when they become unable to make decisions for themselves as has been been shown in other areas of social work practice [23]. As members of interdisciplinary teams, social workers are trained and skilled in providing supportive palliative and end of life care perhaps for extended periods of time, because of advancements in medical technology, rising rates of chronic illness, increasing number of elderly people, and longer life spans [32].

The practice standards for social workers are designed to enhance their cultural awareness and maintaining skills, knowledge, values, methods, and sensitivities needed to provide whole-person care with attention to the individual family and often, their health care team members and the community as culturally preferred [20, 32]. The exploration of emotional intelligence (EI) within hospice, palliative and end-of-life care settings underscores its critical role in improving patient outcomes, fostering better interpersonal relationships among healthcare providers, and enhancing stress management capabilities. The integration of EI training, particularly through the involvement of social workers, presents a promising strategy to address these aspects comprehensively. Scholarship has explored the correlation between emotional intelligence and patient satisfaction. The positive correlation between high EI in medical professionals and increased patient satisfaction is evident. Studies consistently demonstrate that empathetic healthcare providers can better understand and meet patient needs, which enhances the overall patient experience [5]. For instance, empathy allows healthcare providers to connect with patients on a personal level, fostering trust and a deeper therapeutic alliance [5]. Patients who feel understood and valued are more likely to report higher satisfaction levels, which can lead to better adherence to treatment plans and improved health outcomes [6].

5. Emotional intelligence and interpersonal relationships

Interpersonal relationships among healthcare providers are crucial for effective patient care. High EI facilitates better teamwork, as emotionally intelligent professionals can navigate the complex social dynamics within healthcare teams. They are more adept at managing conflicts and understanding their colleagues' perspectives, which promotes a collaborative and supportive work environment. For members of the care team, this collaborative culture not only improves job satisfaction but also enhances the overall quality of care provided to patients [24].

Emotional intelligence (EI) and stress management have a level of intersectionality that social workers are prepared to address effective [32]. The ability to manage stress is learned professional behavior for social workers, demonstratives of effectiveness high-pressure health care environments. EI is a tool that enables prepares clinicians to recognize and regulate their emotions under stress in the face of loss and constant incurable disease for patients and families, helping them maintain strength, perseverance to remain focused on the best possible care options and resilience in the face of challenges [34]. Furthermore, when patient experiences anxiety related to a serious illness, or other health anxiety or illness anxiety when living with an incurable disease, it may be worthwhile to consider EI as a strategy to address such challenges, in a controlled environment when communication is not a physical limitation, but may be a mental health limitation for the patient, as has been recommended in literature with other populations [25]. Furthermore, emotionally intelligent clinicians in serious illness care can support their patients, families and colleagues, creating a more supportive and less stressful work environment. This improved stress management can lead to reduced burnout and improved overall well-being for health care professionals, ultimately benefiting patient care [25].

Social workers have documented that essential assessment tools and approaches to social justice, equity and diversity are important to patient and families [18, 32]. Furthermore, social workers strive to enhance emotional intelligence on the respective serious illness care teams [16]. Social workers, with their training in empathy, ethical decision-making, and emotional regulation, are uniquely positioned to lead EI initiatives in healthcare settings. By training and advising interdisciplinary teams about how to develop the essential EI for seriously ill patients and families, social workers can demonstrate skills and impart essential knowledge about how to recognize and manage emotions, improving communication, and building empathy. Moreover, social workers can provide ongoing support and mentorship, helping healthcare providers apply EI principles in their daily practice [29]. This continuous professional development ensures that clinicians engage in continuing education to remain proficient in EI skills and adapt to the evolving needs of their patients [5].

6. Future directions

Hospice, palliative and end-of-life care practitioners, educators, students, and researchers can benefit from the current knowledge that helps to close the gap in understanding and practice approaches to caring for culturally diverse patients and families. Based on the findings of this review of scholarly literature to address the specific questions that can guide future work in EI with seriously ill patients, research should focus on several key areas to further understand and optimize the integration of EI in hospice, palliative and end-of-life care. Longitudinal studies [35] could lead to important findings. Conducting clinical trials and longitudinal studies to assess the long-term impact of EI training on patient outcomes and healthcare provider well-being. Such studies can provide valuable insights into the sustainability and effectiveness of EI interventions over time. To evaluate various work environments, interdisciplinary approaches could contribute to new understanding. Exploring interdisciplinary approaches that involve not only social workers but also psychologists, counselors, and other mental health professionals in EI training and support initiatives. This comprehensive approach can enhance the overall effectiveness of EI programs in healthcare settings.

Technology integration has the potential to uncover new pathways to explore. Investigating the use of technology, such as virtual reality and mobile applications, to deliver EI training and support can broaden the capacity of EI training [13]. These tools can provide scalable and accessible solutions for continuous EI development among healthcare providers. Technology along with policy development can offer new frameworks for how to explore EI training. Advocating for policy changes that recognize the importance of EI in healthcare and support the integration of EI training into medical education and professional development programs. Policies should also address the need for adequate resources and support palliative care systems to sustain EI initiatives. Policy development should include patient perspectives. Including patient perspectives in research can offer ways to understand how EI among hospice, palliative and end-of-life care providers influences their experiences and outcomes. This patient-centered approach can provide valuable insights into the specific needs and preferences of patients regarding emotional care.

A decade of research points to educating and preparing future generations of culturally diverse serious illness clinicians and researchers is an important step to take as well [36, 37]. By addressing these areas, future research can contribute to a deeper understanding of the role of EI in serious illness care also, and inform the development of effective strategies to enhance EI among interdisciplinary teams of professionals, ultimately leading to better patient care and improved healthcare provider well-being.

7. Conclusion

The integration of emotional intelligence (EI) within hospice, palliative and end-of-life care settings, especially through the education and preparation of social workers, presents a significant opportunity to enhance patient care, improve clinician/ provider well-being, and foster better interpersonal relationships between patient/families and health care teams. Previous research emphasizes the need for EI in healthcare professionals, which can lead to increased patient satisfaction, stronger team dynamics, and improved stress management are well-supported by existing research [38]. Empirical research is warranted to test hypotheses about such associations and causation [4]. However, in the meantime, what we know from the scholarly evidence is that social workers, with their specialized training in empathy and ethical decision-making, are ideally prepared to spearhead EI initiatives in serious illness care environments.

The research clearly indicates that emotionally intelligent (EI) health care providers can better understand and meet patient needs, leading to higher patient satisfaction [35]. Empathy, a core component of EI, give providers the capacity to connect with patients on a personal level, fostering trust and a deeper therapeutic relationship [11, 38]. As patients feel more understood and valued, they are more likely to adhere to treatment plans, resulting in better health outcomes.

Effective patient care relies heavily on strong interpersonal relationships within healthcare teams. High EI enables healthcare providers to navigate complex social dynamics, manage conflicts, and understand colleagues' perspectives, promoting a collaborative and supportive work environment [11]. This improved teamwork not only enhances job satisfaction but also the quality of care delivered to patients.

In serious illness care settings, the ability to manage stress is crucial. The skill and knowledge of EI equips health care providers with the skills to recognize and regulate their emotions, maintaining composure and resilience during challenging situations. This is much needed in hospice, palliative and end-of-life care.

Furthermore, emotionally intelligent professionals can offer better support to their colleagues, reducing overall stress levels and preventing burnout, which ultimately benefits patient care.

Social workers, with their expertise in empathy, ethical practice, and emotional regulation, are uniquely positioned to lead EI initiatives in healthcare. They can train and advise medical professionals on essential EI skills, provide ongoing support, and help healthcare providers apply EI principles in their daily practice [20, 38]. This continuous professional development ensures that healthcare providers remain proficient in EI, adapting to the evolving needs of their patients [12]. By focusing on these research areas can contribute to a deeper understanding of EI's role in healthcare, informing the development of effective strategies to enhance EI among healthcare professionals. This, in turn, will lead to better patient care and improved well-being for healthcare providers.

Author details

Terrance Ruth
School of Social Work and Africana Studies, NC State University, Raleigh, USA

*Address all correspondence to: trruth@ncsu.edu

References

[1] Ruth TR, Bullock K, O'Conner K, Anderson G. Emotional intelligence and clinician empathy: An interdisciplinary model for understanding and addressing clinician disruptive behavior. International Journal of Humanities and Social Science. 2024;**14**(1):182-192

[2] Ironside PM. Exploring the complexity of advocacy: Balancing patient-centered care and safety. Nursing Outlook. 2008;**57**(6):338-3482

[3] Bullock K. The influence of culture on end-of-life decision making. In: Partners in Palliative Care. Routledge; 2013. pp. 82-97

[4] Ruth T, Matusitz J. Comparative standards of evidence in social work. Journal of Evidence-Based Social Work. 2013;**10**(4):285-298

[5] Pérez-Fuentes MD, Molero Jurado MD, Del Pino RM, Gázquez Linares JJ. Emotional intelligence, self-efficacy and empathy as predictors of overall self-esteem in nursing by years of experience. Frontiers in Psychology. 2019;**18**(10):1-9

[6] Weng H-C. Does the physician's emotional intelligence matter?: Impacts of the physician's emotional intelligence on the trust, patient-physician relationship, and satisfaction. Health Care Management Review. 2008;**33**(4):280-288

[7] Jain S. In Search of the Art of Healing in Modern Medicine. 2006. Available from: https://journalofethics.ama-assn.org/article/search-art-healing-modern-medicine/2006-07

[8] Colomer-Sánchez A, Ayuso-Murillo D, Lendínez-Mesa A, Ruiz-Nuñez C, Fontán-Vinagre G, Herrera-Peco I. Anxiety effect on communication skills in nursing supervisors: An observational study. Nursing Reports. 2021;**11**(2):207-216

[9] Finset A. Emotional intelligence, alexithymia, and the doctor-patient relationship. In: Koh K, editor. Somatization and Psychosomatic Symptoms. New York, NY: Springer; 2013

[10] Starr LT, Bullock K, Washington K, Aryal S, Parker Oliver D, Demiris G. Anxiety, depression, quality of life, caregiver burden, and perceptions of caregiver-centered communication among black and white hospice family caregivers. Journal of Palliative Medicine. 2022;**25**(4):596-605

[11] Taylor J, Fradgley EA, Clinton-McHarg T, Hall A, Paul CL. Perceived importance of emotional support provided by health care professionals and social networks: Should we broaden our focus for the delivery of supportive care? Asia Pacific Journal of Clinical Oncology. 2023;**19**(6):681-689

[12] Petrova E, Dewing J, Camilleri M. Confidentiality in participatory research: Challenges from one study. Nursing Ethics. 2016;**23**(4):442-454

[13] Quinn JF, Hoffe SE. The Importance of Emotional Intelligence in Healthcare. 2014. Available from: https://www.healthcatalyst.com/insights/emotional-intelligence-healthcare

[14] Wiechula R, Conroy T, Kitson AL, Marshall RJ, Whitaker N, Rasmussen P. Umbrella review of the evidence: What factors influence the caring relationship between a nurse and patient? Journal of Advanced Nursing. 2016;**72**(4):723-734

[15] Dobrofa J, Craig SL, Ferruzzi L. Innovations in efficient, effective and quality oriented practices and procedures in healthcare social work. Social Work in Health Care. 2024;**63**(4-5):205-2071

[16] Bullock K, Bullock-Johnson R. Cultural humility: Necessary but insufficient for equitable access to care. In: Doka KJ, Jennings B, Kirk TW, Tucci AS, editors. End-of-Life Ethics in a Changing World. Washington, DC: Hospice Foundation of America Press; 2023. pp. 73-85

[17] Bullock K, Gray TF, Tucker R, Quest TE. Race roundtable series: Structural racism in palliative care. Journal of Pain and Symptom Management. 2022b;**S0885-3924**(22):00038. DOI: 10.1016/j.jpainsymman.2022.01.015

[18] Wallace CL, Subramaniam DS, Wray R, Bullock K, Dant D, Coccia K, et al. Development of a hospice perceptions instrument for diverse patients and families: Establishing content and face validity. The American Journal of Hospice & Palliative Care. 2024:1-8

[19] Rhodes R, Ejem D, Barrett N, Smith C, Bullock K, Bethea K, et al. Association and causation without adequate representation: An evaluation of the reporting of race and ethnicity of study participants in hospice and palliative medicine research (GP751). Journal of Pain and Symptom Management. 2022;**63**(6):1140. DOI: 10.1016/j.jpainsymman.2022.04.142

[20] Ruth T, Matusitz J. Comparative standards of evidence in social work. Journal of Evidence-Based Social Work. 2010;**10**(4):285-298. DOI: 10.1080/15433714.2012.663660

[21] Butler L, Park SK, Vyas D, Cole JD, Haney JS, Marrs JC, et al. Evidence and strategies for including emotional intelligence in pharmacy education. American Journal of Pharmaceutical Education. 2022;**86**(10):ajpe8674. DOI: 10.5688/ajpe8674

[22] Salovey P, Mayer JD. Emotional intelligence. Imagination, Cognition and Personality. 1990;**9**(3):185-211

[23] Ruth T, O'Connor K. The role of social work in integrating mental health students in traditional school settings: Community care approach. Journal of Mental Health & Social Behavior. 2020;**2**(1):119. DOI: 10.33790/jmhsb1100119

[24] James TA. The Power of Emotional Intelligence in the Doctor-Patient Relationship. 2023. Available from: https://etsdental.com/the-power-of-emotional-intelligence-in-the-doctor-patient-relationship/

[25] Archbell KA, Coplan RJ. Too anxious to talk: Social anxiety, academic communication, and students' experiences in higher education. Journal of Emotional and Behavioral Disorders. 2022;**30**(4):273-286. DOI: 10.1177/10634266211060079

[26] Miotto K, Sanford J, Brymer MJ, Bursch B, Pynoos RS. Implementing an emotional support and mental health response plan for healthcare workers during the COVID-19 pandemic. Psychological Trauma: Theory, Research, Practice and Policy. 2020;**12**(S1):S165-S167

[27] Morrison J. The relationship between emotional intelligence competencies and preferred conflict-handling styles. Journal of Nursing Management. 2008;**16**(8):974-983

[28] Sosin M, Caulum S. Advocacy: A conceptualization for social work practice. Social Work. 1983;**28**(1):12-17

[29] Health Catalyst. The Importance of Emotional Intelligence in Healthcare. 2020. Available from: https://www.healthcatalyst.com/insights/emotional-intelligence-healthcare

[30] Csikai EL, Bullock K. The growth of social work in palliative and end-of-life care in the United States: How did we get here? Palliative Care and Social Practice. 2024;**18**:26323524241263625

[31] American Medical Association. How Emotional Intelligence Can Improve Patient Care. 2021. Available from: https://www.ama-assn.org/delivering-care/patient-support-advocacy/how-emotional-intelligence-can-improve-patient-care

[32] National Association of Social Workers. Standards for Palliative and End-of-Life Care. Washington, DC: NASW Author; 2015

[33] Anderson G, Bullock K, Fitzpatrick DF, Ruth TR. Cultural competence, emotional intelligence and social work practice. InterSections in Practice. 2021;**15**:34-35

[34] Rosa WE, Ahmed E, Chaila MJ, Chansa A, Cordoba MA, Dowla R, et al. Can you hear us now? Equity in global advocacy for palliative care. Journal of Pain and Symptom Management. 2022;**64**(4):e217-e226

[35] Wasfie T, Kirkpatrick H, Barber K, HellaJR, AndersonT, VogelM. Longitudinal study of emotional intelligence, well-being, and burnout of surgical and medical residents. The American Surgeon. 2023;**89**(7):3077-3083. DOI: 10.1177/00031348231157813

[36] Smith AK, Thai JN, Bakitas MA, Meier DE, Spragens LH, Temel JS, et al. The diverse landscape of palliative care clinics. Journal of Palliative Medicine. 2013;**16**(6):661-668. DOI: 10.1089/jpm.2012.0469

[37] Zehm A, Smith S, Schaefer KG, Jonas D, Bullock K, et al. Development of objectives to inform a national standardized primary palliative care curriculum for health professions students. Journal of Palliative Medicine. 2023;**26**(3):406-410

[38] Hilas O. Empathy or empath? Increasing self-awareness for healthy patient-provider interactions. The Senior Care Pharmacist. 2020;**35**(8):334-335. DOI: 10.4140/TCP.n.2020.334

Chapter 3

Perspective Chapter: Palliative Care for Patients with Chronic Kidney Disease in Low-Resource Settings

Sserusiba Hassan

Abstract

CKD is a significant public health concern due to its high incidence, prevalence, and impact on morbidity, mortality, and socioeconomic burdens. Over 10% of the global population is affected, with approximately 843.6 million cases in 2017. In Sub-Saharan Africa, the CKD prevalence ranges from 10 to 13%, with 6.8% in East Africa. Factors like hypertension, diabetes, and delayed diagnosis contribute to the increasing CKD burden in the region. In low-resource settings, CKD patients face substantial morbidity and mortality, with severe physical symptoms, emotional distress, and psychosocial challenges worsened by limited specialized care. CKD is often detected late, shifting the focus from curative treatments to the improvement of quality of life. Dialysis, a common therapeutic intervention, often lowers the overall quality of life and functional status, with cessation linked to high mortality rates. Many patients stop dialysis near the end-of-life, necessitating comprehensive palliative care. Despite the rising demand, access to palliative care for CKD patients is limited. Palliative care aims to alleviate suffering and enhance quality of life through pain and symptom management, as well as psychosocial and spiritual support. This chapter examines CKD patients' unique palliative care needs, challenges faced by patients, families, and healthcare providers in low-resource settings, and strategies to incorporate palliative care into the national healthcare system for a holistic approach to chronic disease management.

Keywords: chronic kidney disease (CKD), palliative care, low-resource settings, symptom management, low- and middle-income countries (LMICs)

1. Introduction

Chronic kidney disease (CKD) is a progressive condition that affects approximately 13% of the global population and often leads to end-stage renal disease (ESRD) [1–13]. Chronic kidney disease (CKD) is defined by the presence of kidney damage or an estimated glomerular filtration rate (eGFR) of less than 60 mL/min/1.73 m^2, persisting for a duration of three months or longer. This condition is characterized by a progressive decline in kidney function, which frequently necessitates renal replacement therapy, such as dialysis or kidney transplantation [14]. Chronic kidney disease (CKD) is a significant public health concern because of its high incidence, prevalence, and impact on morbidity and mortality rates and associated socioeconomic burdens, particularly in low- and middle-income countries (LMICs) [1, 15].

Globally, the prevalence of chronic kidney disease (CKD) is rapidly increasing, with an estimated 843.6 million people affected [2, 3]. This rising prevalence is attributed to various factors such as diabetes, hypertension, obesity, high infectious disease rates, and exposure to environmental toxins [16]. Additionally, chronic infections, such as HIV, hepatitis B, and hepatitis C, along with the widespread utilization of herbal medications in low-income settings, significantly exacerbate the prevalence of CKD [17]. LMICs encounter distinct obstacles in addressing CKD, including limited healthcare resources, limited health insurance coverage, and predominant out-of-pocket expenditure on medical care [15]. It is estimated that 434.3 million adults in Asia have chronic kidney disease (CKD). China and India have the highest number of adults living with CKD, with estimates reaching up to 159.8 million and 140.2 million individuals respectively, accounting for 69.1% of the total number of adults with CKD in the region [18]. In Sub-Saharan Africa, the estimated proportion of individuals presumed to have kidney disease ranges from 10 to 13% [4]. The overall prevalence of chronic kidney disease (CKD) in East Africa is estimated at 6.8%, with regional variations of 12.5% in eastern Uganda, 3.9% in southwestern Uganda, and 3.7% in western Kenya [5].

Patients with advanced CKD have decreased life expectancy and experience significant morbidity and mortality, as evidenced by a study that reported an average of 10.5 symptoms in severely ill individuals [6]. Distressing symptoms include pain, fatigue, sleep disorders, itching, nausea, shortness of breath, anxiety, and depression [7]. Failure to address these symptoms in patients with chronic kidney disease can result in a low quality of life, characterized by pain, discomfort, and distress. Healthcare professionals must possess advanced knowledge of pain and symptom management, accompanied by effective communication skills, to address the diverse needs of this population [19].

Palliative care is increasingly recognized as essential for patients suffering from chronic kidney disease (CKD) and end-stage renal disease (ESRD), who may lack access to curative or life-prolonging treatments, as it addresses their high symptom burden, reduces healthcare costs by preventing unnecessary hospital admissions, and improves their overall quality of life [20, 21]. This approach is especially critical in low-resource settings, where palliative interventions can help alleviate pain, address multifaceted symptoms such as uremic pruritus and dyspnea, and provide support for patients and their families in managing the adversities of progressive illness [22]. However, the integration of palliative care in LMICs for CKD management faces barriers, including financial limitations, scarcity of healthcare professionals, restricted access to specialized services, underdeveloped care models, insufficient policy frameworks, competing healthcare priorities, and lack of awareness regarding palliative care needs, all of which contribute to inadequate support for CKD patients [21]. To overcome these challenges, a collaborative approach involving primary care, nephrology, and palliative care specialists is recommended [23]. Various palliative care approaches, such as conservative management, peritoneal dialysis, and extracorporeal palliative dialysis, can be tailored to meet the physical, social, psychological, and spiritual needs of patients [24].

This chapter explores the landscape of palliative care for CKD patients in low-resource settings, examining the scope of palliative care for patients with CKD, barriers to access, and potential strategies to improve care.

2. Burden of chronic kidney disease in low and middle-income countries (LMICs)

Globally, the estimated prevalence of patients with ESRD requiring renal replacement therapy (RRT) ranges from 4.902 to 9.701 million, with the majority of these cases occurring in LMICs [25]. The accessibility to kidney replacement therapy (KRT) is limited globally, with less than half of those in need being able to obtain it. The disparity between high-income countries (HICs) and low-income countries (LICs) is stark. In LMICs, KRT remains inaccessible for up to 98% of individuals with kidney failure, whereas in HICs, it drops to 30%. Notably, 88% of the patients lacking access to KRT are located in African or Asian nations [26].

The burden of chronic kidney disease (CKD) is particularly high in resource-limited settings, especially in Africa, and is attributed to increased exposure to infections, poverty, poor accessibility to healthcare services, and genetic predispositions [27]. While middle-aged and elderly populations are predominantly affected in developed nations, in Sub-Saharan Africa, CKD predominantly affects young adults during their economically productive years, with hypertension and infection-related chronic glomerulonephritis identified as the major etiological causes. The morbidity and mortality associated with CKD are significantly higher in LMICs because of the inability of most affected individuals to access renal replacement therapy [28]. A 2017 Global Burden of Disease study revealed that CKD was responsible for approximately 1.2 million deaths globally, with over two-thirds of these deaths occurring in LMICs [29]. In these regions, the overwhelming majority of patients lack access to renal replacement therapy, and the scarcity of resources has impeded the widespread utilization of prevention strategies [27, 30].

The prevalence of chronic kidney disease (CKD) and end-stage kidney disease (ESKD) constitutes significant public health challenges in LMICs, where the limited availability of treatment options contributes to elevated mortality rates. Despite reports indicating a lower overall prevalence, a larger proportion of CKD patients in LMICs lack effective treatment than those in high-income countries [31]. Economic and health system constraints create significant inequities in access to kidney replacement therapies including dialysis and transplantation [31, 32]. Notably, only 12% of low-income countries provide kidney transplantation services [31].

The financial burden associated with the management of CKD grows exponentially as the disease advances, with annual expenditures per patient ranging from $3500 for CKD stage 3 to over $50,000 when kidney failure occurs, necessitating kidney replacement therapy. In many wealthy nations, these expenses are mitigated through Medicare reimbursements and/or universal health insurance programs. However, in many LMICs, the lack of protection against catastrophic health expenditures has led to a heightened dependence on out-of-pocket health expenditures, thereby exposing patients and their families to significant financial jeopardy and potentially relegating them to extreme poverty as a consequence of medical expenses [33, 34].

The absence of kidney registries in numerous LMICs poses significant challenges for accurately determining the prevalence of CKD [35]. Healthcare practitioners operating within resource-limited settings often fail to adequately identify and manage CKD and its associated risk factors at the primary care level. Furthermore, the recognition and management of acute kidney injury (AKI) is markedly inadequate, leading to delayed nephrologist referrals and increased mortality rates. Sociocultural factors and economic hardships prevalent in low-income regions exacerbate and contribute to the late presentation of kidney disease [36]. Additionally, limited health literacy among the population and reliance on alternative healthcare practices, including herbal remedies, may further hinder the timely diagnosis of kidney disease. These alternative treatments can potentially cause AKI and accelerate its progression to renal failure [37].

In low-income settings, the ratio of nephrologists to the population is markedly lower, with only 0.31 nephrologists per million population, compared to high-income countries that have 28.5 per million [38]. This shortage of nephrology specialists in resource-constrained settings results in suboptimal management of renal diseases and potentially fewer public health initiatives aimed at preventing and managing them [17].

Addressing the challenges involved in the management of CKD in LMICs necessitates a multifaceted approach encompassing community engagement, awareness campaigns, and screening programs [17]. In areas with limited resources, where serum creatinine measurements may not be available, a basic CKD screening program could integrate tests for proteinuria, blood glucose, blood pressure, and body mass index. Substantial efforts are essential to augment resources and improve access to affordable renal replacement therapy options in the coming decades [30]. However, financial limitations impede these efforts. Prevention strategies should prioritize education, early detection, and lifestyle changes [35]. Utilizing task-shifting approaches and enhancing the capabilities of primary healthcare providers can contribute to improved CKD prevention and management in resource-constrained settings [17].

3. Scope of palliative care in CKD management

Palliative care in chronic kidney disease (CKD) extends far beyond end-of-life care, offering a patient-centered approach that emphasizes improving quality of life, managing complex symptoms, and providing holistic support to patients and their families. The integration of palliative care into CKD management is critical, especially in low-resource settings where access to life-prolonging treatments such as dialysis and kidney transplantation is limited (Murtagh et al., 2011). This section explores the multidimensional scope of palliative care within the CKD continuum.

3.1 Symptom management

Patients with CKD frequently experience a wide range of distressing symptoms, encompassing pain, uremic pruritus, dyspnea, fatigue, muscle cramps, nausea, vomiting, and anorexia, which significantly diminish their quality of life. Although these symptoms are prevalent among patients suffering from other advanced chronic illnesses such as cancer and congestive heart failure. Palliative care provides evidence-based strategies to alleviate these symptoms, focusing on both pharmacological and non-pharmacological interventions. For example, pain management protocols tailored to CKD patients address renal-safe analgesics and dosage adjustments to minimize toxicity [39, 40].

Fatigue, frequently associated with decreased oxygen delivery, lactic acidosis, chronic metabolic acidosis, protein-energy wasting, hyperphosphatemia, depression, and anemia, is one of the most frequently reported symptoms among CKD patients, with prevalence rates ranging from 20 to 91%. The palliative care approach for patients with fatigue begins with a thorough assessment of the underlying causes, which includes the identification and management of anemia, sleep disturbances, and depression [41].

Pain, which can be (neuropathic, nociceptive, or both), is another prevalent symptom. The occurrence of moderate to severe pain is particularly high, significantly affecting daily functioning and overall quality of life. In LMICs, where resources for pain management are scarce, this symptom often remains poorly addressed. Untreated pain in this population negatively impacts health-related quality of life (HRQOL), dialysis adherence, healthcare utilization, and mortality and may also exacerbate other physical and psychosocial symptoms such as depression, anxiety, and fatigue [40, 42].

Effective pain management in patients with CKD requires a comprehensive assessment process. This process includes: (1) quantifying pain intensity using standardized tools, such as the numerical rating scale, (2) conducting a pathophysiological examination to determine the pain's origin and type, (3) assessing psychosocial factors that may exacerbate pain or complicate its treatment, such as depression, anxiety, and (4) Evaluating the overall impact of pain on the patient's quality of life using validated instruments like the PEG (Pain average, interference with Enjoyment of life, and interference with general activity) [40].

A decline in glomerular filtration rate (GFR) significantly influences the standard pharmacokinetics of analgesic medications, increasing the likelihood of toxicity, undesirable side effects, and drug interactions. The effective management of patients with reduced GFR necessitates careful analgesic selection, dose titration, and monitoring. Non-pharmacological approaches, including physical therapy and relaxation techniques, can complement pharmacological treatments and enhance symptom relief [43].

Chronic kidney disease-associated pruritus, also known as uremic pruritus, is a severely distressing condition often underdiagnosed, affecting approximately 60% of patients undergoing dialysis. It also occurs in non-dialysis patients with stages 3–5 CKD, with prevalence increasing with the decline in renal function, advancing age, and the presence of comorbidities [44]. Effective management includes optimizing dialysis, using phosphate binders, phototherapy, skin hydration with emollients, tacrolimus ointment, and capsaicin creams, along with the utilization of pharmacological agents such as gabapentin or pregabalin and antihistamines [45].

Nausea, characterized as an unpleasant sensation associated with the imminent urge to vomit, may manifest either independently or in conjunction with vomiting, dyspepsia, or other gastrointestinal symptoms, with a prevalence in CKD patients ranging from 30 to 43%. The etiology of nausea is multifactorial, often associated with metabolic or gastrointestinal disturbances and medication side effects, which become more common as kidney disease advances. Ondansetron is recommended as the first-line treatment for nausea and vomiting in CKD patients. Other medications used included metoclopramide and olanzapine. Including dietary modifications and complementary interventions such as massage, guided imagery, and music therapy, are recommended because of the side effects frequently associated with common pharmacological medications [39].

Holistic palliative care strategies, including patient education, dietary interventions, and psychological support, are crucial in addressing these physical symptoms in patients with CKD in LMICs, where there are limited resources, especially palliative care medicines, for effective management of these symptoms in order to improve their quality of life but also foster better adherence to treatment regimens.

3.2 Psychosocial and emotional support

Adjustment after the diagnosis of a chronic disease presents considerable psychosocial and emotional challenges. Patients diagnosed with chronic kidney disease (CKD) are no exception as they are compelled to undertake continuous psychological adjustments, which include the acceptance of a life-threatening condition, adherence to lifelong therapeutic regimens, learning dialysis techniques, integrating treatment into daily lives, and management of treatment transitions, failures, adverse effects, and complications [46].

Patients with CKD frequently experience psychological distress, including depression, anxiety, and stress, which significantly impact their quality of life. Studies have shown that CKD patients exhibit higher levels of depression and anxiety compared to healthy individuals [47, 48]. The prevalence of clinically significant depression, anxiety, health anxiety, and sleep disturbance in non-dialysis CKD patients was found to be 3.1%, 3.1%, 18%, and 36.2%, respectively [49].

Studies in LMICs have revealed a high prevalence of psychosocial distress among patients with CKD. Studies in Sri Lanka and Nigeria revealed that 75% and 65.2% of CKD patients, respectively, experienced psychological distress, with notable correlations with advanced age, unemployment, and poor health-related quality of life [50, 51]. Furthermore, another study indicated that 55.2% of CKD patients reported experiencing psychological distress, which was associated with factors such as poor social support, financial instability, and female gender [52].

The nature of psychological distress in CKD is inherently multidimensional, encompassing depression, anxiety, stress, and panic, resulting from a complex interplay of biological, psychological, spiritual, and socioeconomic factors [53]. Notably, the severity of psychological symptoms does not significantly differ across CKD stages [49]. These findings highlight the critical importance of addressing the psychosocial and emotional concerns among CKD patients and emphasize the need for a holistic approach to patient care [48].

Patients with CKD in low- and middle-income countries (LMICs) encounter unique psychosocial and emotional challenges that emerge from socioeconomic disparities and limited healthcare resources. Financial insecurity is a significant contributor to distress, as a majority of patients in LMICs are required to pay out-of-pocket for diagnostic tests, medications, and treatments like dialysis [16, 54]. The exorbitant costs associated with these services often lead to treatment delays or discontinuation, thereby exacerbating the psychological burden of living with a progressive illness. Moreover, the absence of universal health coverage or social support programs further exacerbates feelings of helplessness and vulnerability among patients and their families [55, 56].

The cultural stigma associated with chronic illnesses in LMICs also distinctly affects patients with CKD. In some communities, CKD may be perceived as a punishment for previous transgressions or a sign of weakness, leading to social isolation and discrimination. This stigma is particularly pronounced in rural areas where knowledge about CKD is low. Additionally, inadequate healthcare infrastructure frequently necessitates long-distance travel to access specialized care, thereby causing physical exhaustion and emotional stress. The limited access to mental health services in LMICs further limits patients' access to psychosocial support services, leaving many to cope with anxiety and depression in solitude [50, 57, 58].

In low- and middle-income countries (LMICs), a palliative care approach aimed at addressing psychosocial and emotional distress in CKD necessitates an examination of the interplay between resource limitations, stigma, and cultural dynamics. Empirical evidence indicates that the integration of psychosocial care into CKD management improves mental health outcomes and patient satisfaction, even in resource-constrained environments [59]. For example, community health workers trained in basic counseling skills have effectively provided mental health support in LMICs, mitigating depression and anxiety among patients with chronic illnesses [60].

Peer support groups, especially those that capitalize on shared experiences, have been shown to alleviate social isolation and promote emotional resilience [58]. Financial assistance programs, often implemented through partnerships with nongovernmental organizations, have demonstrated effectiveness in alleviating the economic burden associated with CKD management, thereby facilitating improved adherence to treatment and reducing associated distress [61]. Additionally, culturally tailored interventions, such as collaborations with religious and community leaders, have been effective in combating illness-related stigma and providing spiritual support, which holds particular significance in LMIC contexts [62]. These strategies, anchored within a palliative care framework, holistically address the psychological and emotional needs of CKD patients, demonstrating a pragmatic and evidence-based approach to care delivery in low-resource environments.

3.3 Spiritual support in CKD

In low- and middle-income countries (LMICs), the phenomenon of spiritual distress experienced by patients with CKD is profoundly influenced by cultural and socioeconomic factors. Many patients view CKD as a punishment for previous transgressions or a spiritual trial, leading to guilt, shame, and existential despair, particularly when coupled with financial hardships and limited access to medical care. Research indicates that unresolved spiritual issues, including the fear of death or questioning the purpose of suffering, substantially exacerbate emotional distress and reduce overall quality of life [62, 63]. Despite the absence of structured spiritual care services in most LMIC healthcare systems, faith-based organizations and religious leaders frequently intervene to deliver essential support through prayers, rituals, and culturally attuned guidance, thereby providing patients with a sense of purpose and hope [64].

However, conflicting messages from traditional healers or faith leaders regarding medical interventions sometimes create barriers to access to healthcare highlighting the necessity of integrating spiritual care into the management of CKD. Evidence suggests that training healthcare providers to address spiritual needs and fostering collaborations with faith leaders can significantly reduce spiritual distress and improve patient outcomes in LMICs. Acknowledging and addressing the spiritual dimensions of CKD promotes a holistic approach to care that supports patients and their families throughout the disease trajectory, particularly during end-of-life stages [58, 65, 66].

3.4 Advance care planning and decision-making

Advance care planning is an important element of palliative care, with its significance evolving from an exclusive focus on patients at the terminal stage of life to its applicability across all stages of illness. The primary objective of advanced care planning is to prepare patients with diverse health conditions to make informed treatment choices [67]. Advance care planning is recommended for patients with chronic kidney disease alongside their families, which is beneficial throughout the disease trajectory. In low- and middle-income countries (LMICs), the provision of advance care planning (ACP) and decision-making support for CKD patients is imperative, given the unique challenges they encounter such as financial constraints, limited access to dialysis and transplantation, and deficient palliative care services [68, 69].

Patients and their families frequently face difficult decisions regarding the continuation of expensive treatments such as dialysis, often grappling with financial implications in contrast to potential advantages, typically without sufficient guidance [4]. Cultural traditions in LMICs, where healthcare decisions are frequently collective and family-centered, require ACP approaches that honor these dynamics while prioritizing patient autonomy [67]. The presence of low health literacy, limited awareness, unrealistic expectations or hopes for a cure, and limited understanding of CKD progression and advance care planning among healthcare professionals, patients, and their caretakers further hinders informed decision-making, emphasizing the need for early and ongoing communication about treatment goals, prognosis, and end-of-life care options [70]. Evidence suggests that integrating culturally sensitive communication techniques, training healthcare providers in ACP, and the engagement of religious leaders or traditional healers in discussions can enhance the acceptance of care plans and ensure alignment with patients' values and preferences [71]. These interventions are vital for enabling informed and compassionate decision-making in resource-constrained settings.

Palliative care serves to facilitate discussions surrounding patient goals, values, and preferences for care, particularly in instances where curative treatments are not feasible. Advance care planning (ACP) allows patients and their families to make informed decisions regarding treatment options, including the option to decline dialysis treatment or pursue conservative management strategies [72, 73]. In resource-limited contexts where dialysis may be unaffordable or inaccessible, ACP becomes an essential component of compassionate care, enabling informed and compassionate decision-making in resource-limited settings.

3.5 End-of-life care

End-of-life care for renal patients has historically been inadequate, despite a higher incidence of mortality occurring within hospital settings as opposed to that of other patient populations. The necessity of specialist palliative care for patients with advanced chronic kidney disease (CKD) is now acknowledged [74]. The recognition of medical futility, reaching a consensus on it, and the cessation of potentially inappropriate therapeutic interventions represent fundamental initial steps in the provision of end-of-life care. Essential components encompass holding family meetings, communicating prognosis, discussing treatment options, negotiating care goals, shared decision-making, and documentation of preferences regarding life-sustaining interventions.

End-of-life care involves the assessment and management of symptoms associated with end-stage kidney disease while also providing support to families during bereavement [75]. Community-based palliative care models that incorporate multidisciplinary teams, faith leaders, and culturally sensitive communication strategies have demonstrated potential in delivering accessible and compassionate end-of-life care, thereby aligning care with the values of patients and safeguarding their dignity in the dying process. Culturally sensitive approaches are particularly important in diverse low-resource settings where beliefs concerning death and dying may substantially differ [11, 76].

3.6 Support for families and caregivers

Families caring for individuals with chronic kidney disease (CKD) face significant challenges, which include psychological stress, financial strain, and disrupted daily routines [77, 78]. Caregivers, predominantly female family members, often experience significant burdens, psychological distress, and unmet support needs [79].

For families and caregivers of CKD patients in low- and middle-income countries (LMICs), the caregiving burden is often exacerbated by the absence of structured support systems. Families and caregivers frequently find themselves with inadequate information and face discontinuities in care from healthcare professionals, compounded by the psychological burden of indefinite caregiving and uncertainty regarding their loved one's death [80]. Caregivers, typically family members, bear the responsibility of providing daily care, managing medications, and facilitating transportation for treatments such as dialysis, often at considerable personal and economic sacrifices [27].

Financial hardships resulting from healthcare expenditures frequently culminate in debts and strained family relationships, while the emotional toll of caring for a progressively ill loved one contributes to high rates of burnout, anxiety, and depression among caregivers. The limited availability of formal training and counseling services further exacerbates these difficulties, leaving families inadequately prepared to address caregiving demands. Community-based palliative care models that integrate caregiver education, emotional counseling, and spiritual support have evidenced effectiveness in LMICs, providing caregivers with practical skills, emotional resilience, and relief from isolation thereby empowering them to navigate the challenges of caregiving while safeguarding their own well-being [61, 81]. Such initiatives are crucial for enhancing the well-being of caregivers and sustaining effective care for CKD patients in resource-constrained settings.

4. Barriers to palliative care delivery among CKD patients in LMICs

4.1 Limited awareness and misconceptions about palliative care

Limited awareness and widespread misconceptions regarding palliative care impede its delivery to CKD patients in LMICs, where it is frequently misconstrued as being exclusively related to end-of-life services, thereby neglecting its broader role in improving the quality of life, symptom management, and holistic support from early disease stages [21, 82]. Such misinterpretations result in delayed referrals, with CKD patients accessing palliative care only in advanced stages, if they engage with it at all [61]. The general population and healthcare workers frequently demonstrate a lack of knowledge regarding the benefits of palliative care for chronic conditions like CKD, resulting in underutilization and exclusion from routine care. Awareness campaigns predominantly focus on cancer or HIV/AIDS, leaving conditions like CKD unrecognized as deserving of palliative care interventions. Cultural and societal norms in LMICs may stigmatize discussions about death and non-curative treatments, discouraging open conversations among patients, families, and healthcare practitioners [16, 59, 83].

4.2 Shortage of trained healthcare professionals

The limited nephrology workforce in LMICs hinders the development of palliative care, the provision of kidney disease treatment, and facilities for kidney disease management. It is estimated that approximately 7 million people in LMICs die due to the lack of appropriate dialysis facilities. Socioeconomic and geographic factors, along with inadequate technician and healthcare professional training, hinder the establishment of sustainable dialysis and kidney transplant centers [73, 84, 85]. This scarcity uniquely undermines the provision of palliative care for patients with CKD, especially those who may need palliative dialysis [16, 83]. The inadequacy of palliative care training for healthcare providers, who tend to prioritize curative treatment in light of the overwhelming burden posed by other diseases, further exacerbates this issue [61].

The migration of healthcare professionals from LMICs to HICs worsens staff shortages in LMICs, especially in Sub-Saharan Africa [86, 87]. This phenomenon, referred to as "medical brain drain," is driven by the forces of globalization and the capacity of HICs to attract specialists, adversely affecting health services and outcomes in LMICs [86].

To address these pressing challenges, it is imperative to implement health policy reforms, improved education and training, and integrating palliative care into existing health systems [88]. Collaborative care models involving primary care, nephrology, and palliative care specialists may serve to bridge the existing gaps in palliative care for patients with CKD [23]. The development of both primary and specialized kidney palliative care initiatives is essential to address the impacts of advanced kidney disease and optimize patient quality of life [20].

4.3 Economic challenges and high levels of poverty

Economic challenges significantly impede the delivery of kidney care in low- and middle-income countries (LMICs). Out-of-pocket costs for chronic kidney disease (CKD) treatment increase with disease severity, often leading to financial catastrophe for affected families [89]. These costs adversely influence adherence to prescribed medications and dialysis treatment, with poorer households most affected [90]. LMICs face a severe shortage of nephrologists and limited access to diagnostic tools and renal replacement therapy (RRT) [91]. In contrast to high-income nations that predominantly finance RRT through public means and health insurance, LMICs rely heavily on private and out-of-pocket expenditures [91]. The burden of CKD in LMICs is exacerbated by the double burden of communicable and noncommunicable diseases, and inadequate health insurance and welfare programs [15]. The financial costs associate with CKD care are notably high, encompassing expenses related to dialysis, medications, and frequent hospital admissions. In the absence of universal health coverage or robust social safety nets, many patients are unable to afford even basic palliative services. These financial barriers disproportionately affect the poorest populations, exacerbating health inequities and leaving millions without access to

DOI: http://dx.doi.org/10.5772/intechopen.1009237

essential pain relief and symptom management. These financial barriers disproportionately affect the poorest, worsening health inequities and depriving millions of essential pain relief and symptom management. For CKD patients, economic constraints limit access to life-sustaining treatments and holistic palliative care, often leading to preventable suffering. High poverty levels exacerbate these issues by hindering healthcare infrastructure and workforce capabilities in LMICs, where regions often lack well-equipped facilities and trained professionals needed to provide comprehensive palliative care for CKD patients [16, 91].

4.4 Limited access to essential medicines and resources

The provision of palliative care for patients with chronic kidney disease (CKD) in LMICs is greatly affected by limited access to essential palliative care medications such as oral liquid morphine. A survey revealed that only 31% of the respondents had adequate access to essential kidney medications in LICs and LMICs [26]. The barriers include national health policies, funding issues, and resource limitations. Stringent opioid regulations aimed at controlling misuse often result in limited availability for legitimate medical needs, thereby leaving many patients with CKD suffering from unmanaged pain and symptoms. Financial barriers further exacerbate the problem as a considerable number of patients must pay out-of-pocket for medications, making treatment unaffordable for those already grappling with poverty [26, 89].

The absence of essential medications leads to unnecessary suffering and reduced quality of life for patients and their families. In addition, LMICs face severe shortages and limited access to diagnostic tools and renal replacement therapies [91]. Improving access to essential medicines requires a multifaceted approach, which should encompass health policy changes, legislation reform, professional healthcare education, and research specific to LMICs [88]. Potential interventions should focus on improving affordability through universal healthcare, promoting the judicious use of medicines, and strengthening drug production and supply chains [26]. Addressing these challenges is crucial for reducing CKD progression and improving patient quality of life care outcomes in LMICs [33].

4.5 Cultural and societal perceptions

Cultural and societal perceptions significantly influence the accessibility and utilization of palliative care for patients with CKD in LMICs. A major barrier is stigma and misconceptions about palliative care, which is frequently equated with end-of-life care or giving up treatment [92, 93]. This misunderstanding delays referral to palliative care, despite the potential benefits that patients could derive from symptom relief and psychosocial support [36]. Additionally, cultural beliefs about suffering and death, such as the perception of pain as a natural or spiritual trial, impede the pursuit of medical relief [92].

Family-oriented decision-making, which is common in many LMICs, can also hinder the utilization of palliative care, as families may see it as losing hope for recovery [68]. Additionally, religious beliefs and traditional healing practices further shape the perceptions of palliative care. In many LMICs, the dependence on traditional healers or spiritual practices is deeply rooted, prompting patients and families to prefer these methods to biomedical treatments. This dependence often results in a delay in engagement with formal healthcare systems until CKD has progressed to advanced stages [94–96].

4.6 Policy and regulatory barriers

In many LMICs, palliative care is under-prioritized in national health policies, often overshadowed by curative treatments. Regulatory frameworks in these countries restrict access to palliative care resources, including opioids for pain management. Despite bearing a high burden of untreated pain, LMICs consume only a small fraction of global opioids (International Narcotics Control Board) [88, 97]. Concerns over misuse and diversion have led to stringent regulations and bureaucratic hurdles, limiting opioid access and causing unnecessary suffering for CKD patients [20, 26]. The provision of palliative care is hampered by poor policy enforcement and limited accountability in healthcare systems. This neglect results in insufficient funding, infrastructure, and workforce development for palliative services. Governments must prioritize palliative care in health policies, streamline opioid regulations, and expand health insurance to incorporate essential palliative services for CKD patients [21, 82, 97].

5. Future direction of palliative care in CKD patients in LMICs

Addressing the future of palliative care for CKD patients in LMICs necessitates comprehensive, multi-sectorial approaches to surmount current challenges and satisfy the increasing need for comprehensive care. Integrating palliative care policies is essential, necessitating that governments should incorporate palliative care into national healthcare frameworks and develop regulations that enhance its availability and affordability for CKD patients. This initiative should encompass proper resource allocation, healthcare professional education, and ensuring consistent access to essential medications, particularly opioids for pain control while tackling regulatory barriers [21, 61, 98].

Capacity building is another crucial area of focus, emphasizing the development of a skilled palliative care workforce through specialized training programs for healthcare professionals, including nephrologists, allied healthcare professionals, nurses, and community health workers. Multidisciplinary team approaches should be promoted to deliver holistic care tailored to the complex needs of CKD patients. Additionally, public awareness campaigns and healthcare provider education are also crucial to dispel myths about palliative care [20, 23, 99].

The implementation of innovative care delivery methods utilizing community-based care delivery models and telemedicine can improve palliative care accessibility, particularly in rural and underserved regions [100, 101]. Community health workers with basic palliative care training can act as an extension of the healthcare system, offering symptom management, emotional support, and specialist care referrals. Concurrently, telemedicine can reduce barriers to accessing palliative care specialists, facilitating prompt interventions and consultations for CKD patients [102].

Lastly, it is essential to conduct research in the fields of chronic kidney disease and palliative care to establish a robust evidence base that supports the implementation of palliative care for patients with chronic kidney disease (CKD) [11, 24]. Such evidence has the potential to influence policy decisions and resource allocation while adapting care approaches to meet the unique requirements of populations in low- and middle-income countries (LMICs). By focusing on these areas, LMICs can enhance the well-being of CKD patients, ensuring that palliative care becomes a fundamental component of kidney disease treatment.

Author details

Sserusiba Hassan[1,2]

1 Makerere University, Kampala, Uganda

2 Institute of Hospice and Palliative Care in Africa, Kampala, Uganda

*Address all correspondence to: hassanhanic0@gmail.com

References

[1] Prieto-Velasco M, Pdel Pino Y Pino MD, Buades Fuster JM, Hospital LC, Prades RP, Ruiz San Millán JC, et al. Advanced chronic kidney disease units in Spain: A national survey on standards of structure, resources, results and patient safety. Nefrologia (English Ed). 2020;**40**(6):608-622. Available from: https://www.revistanefrologia.com/en-advanced-chronic-kidney-disease-units-articulo-S2013251420301577

[2] Hill NR, Fatoba ST, Oke JL, Hirst JA, O'Callaghan CA, Lasserson DS, et al. Global prevalence of chronic kidney disease - a systematic review and meta-analysis. PLoS One. Jul 6 2016;**11**(7):e0158765. [cited 2023 Nov 5]; DOI: 10.1371/journal.pone.0158765. Available from: https://pubmed.ncbi.nlm.nih.gov/27383068/

[3] Kovesdy CP. Epidemiology of chronic kidney disease: An update 2022. Kidney International. Supplement. 2022;**12**(1):7-11

[4] Kalyesubula R, Brewster U, Kansiime G. Global dialysis perspective: Uganda. Kidney360. 2022;**3**(5):933. Available from: https://pmc/articles/PMC9438417/

[5] Muiru AN, Charlebois ED, Balzer LB, Kwarisiima D, Elly A, Black D, et al. The epidemiology of chronic kidney disease (CKD) in rural East Africa: A population-based study. PLoS One. 2020;**15**(3):e0229649. Available from: https://journals.plos.org/plosone/article?id=10.1371/journal.pone.0229649

[6] Bagasha P, Leng M, Katabira E, Petrova M. Health-related quality of life, palliative care needs and 12-month survival among patients with end stage renal disease in Uganda: Protocol for a mixed methods longitudinal study. BMC Nephrology. 7 Dec 2020;**21**(1):531. DOI: 10.1186/s12882-020-02197-7

[7] Murtagh FE, Addington-Hall J, Higginson IJ. The prevalence of symptoms in end-stage renal disease: A systematic review. Advances in Chronic Kidney Disease. Jan 2007;**14**(1):82-99. DOI: 10.1053/j.ackd.2006.10.001

[8] Aljawadi MH, Babaeer AA, Alghamdi AS, Alhammad AM, Almuqbil MS, Alonazi KF. Quality of life tools among patients on dialysis: A systematic review. Saudi Pharmaceutical Journal. 2024;**32**(3):101958

[9] Imamah NF, Lin HR. Palliative care in patients with end-stage renal disease: a meta synthesis. International Journal of Environmental Research and Public Health [Internet]. 2 Oct 2021;**18**(20):10651. [cited 2024 Jan 17]. DOI: 10.3390/ijerph182010651

[10] Verberne WR, Tom Geers ABM, Jellema WT, Vincent HH, van Delden JJM, Bos WJW. Comparative survival among older adults with advanced kidney disease managed conservatively versus with dialysis. Clinical Journal of the American Society of Nephrology [Internet]. 7 Apr 2016;**11**(4):633-640. [cited 2025 Feb 16]; DOI: 10.2215/CJN.07510715. Epub 2016 Mar 17. Available from: https://pubmed.ncbi.nlm.nih.gov/26988748/

[11] Tamura MK, O'Hare AM, Lin E, Holdsworth LM, Malcolm E, Moss AH. Palliative care disincentives in CKD: Changing policy to improve CKD care. American Journal of Kidney Diseases. 2018;**71**(6):866-873

[12] Dos Santos Tavares AP, da Silveira Santos CG, Tzanno-Martins C, Neto JB,

da Silva AMM, Lotaif L, et al. Kidney supportive care: An update of the current state of the art of palliative care in CKD patients. Brazilian Journal of Nephrology. 2020;**43**(1):74-87. Available from: https://www.scielo.br/j/jbn/a/8W5QdC4H4dxKzjz8RChtD8G/?lang=en

[13] Evans M, Lewis RD, Morgan AR, Whyte MB, Hanif W, Bain SC, et al. A narrative review of chronic kidney disease in clinical practice: Current challenges and future perspectives. Advances in Therapy. 2022;**39**(1):33-43. Available from: https://pubmed.ncbi.nlm.nih.gov/34739697/

[14] Vaidya SR, Aeddula NR. Chronic kidney disease. In: Scientific Basis of Urology. 2nd ed. 2024. pp. 257-264. Available from: https://www.ncbi.nlm.nih.gov/books/NBK535404/

[15] Ulasi II, Awobusuyi O, Nayak S, Ramachandran R, Musso CG, Depine SA, et al. Chronic kidney disease burden in low-resource settings: Regional perspectives. Seminars in Nephrology [Internet]. 1 Sep 2022;**42**(5):151336. DOI: 10.1016/j.semnephrol.2023.151336. [cited 2024 Nov 10]; Epub 2023 Apr 12. Available from: https://pubmed.ncbi.nlm.nih.gov/37058859/

[16] Stanifer JW, Muiru A, Jafar TH, Patel UD. Chronic kidney disease in low- and middle-income countries. Nephrology, Dialysis, Transplantation. 2016;**31**(6):868-874. Available from: https://pubmed.ncbi.nlm.nih.gov/27217391/

[17] Tannor EK, Calice-Silva V. Kidney health for all—Efforts in low-income settings to enhance community engagement, kidney health awareness, and screening. Kidney International Reports. 2021;7(3):359. Available from: https://pmc.ncbi.nlm.nih.gov/articles/PMC8897301/

[18] Liyanage T, Toyama T, Hockham C, Ninomiya T, Perkovic V, Woodward M, et al. Prevalence of chronic kidney disease in Asia: A systematic review and analysis. BMJ Global Health [Internet]. 25 Jan 2022;7(1):e007525. DOI: 10.1136/bmjgh-2021-007525. [cited 2023 Nov 5]; Available from: https://pubmed.ncbi.nlm.nih.gov/35078812/

[19] Fassett RG, Robertson IK, MacE R, Youl L, Challenor S, Bull R. Palliative care in end-stage kidney disease. Nephrology (Carlton). 2011;**16**(1):4-12. Available from: https://pubmed.ncbi.nlm.nih.gov/21175971/

[20] Lam DY, Scherer JS, Brown M, Grubbs V, Schell JO. A conceptual framework of palliative care across the continuum of advanced kidney disease. Clinical Journal of the American Society of Nephrology. 2019;**14**(4):635-641. Available from: https://pubmed.ncbi.nlm.nih.gov/30728167/

[21] Tamura MK, O'Hare AM, Lin E, Holdsworth LM, Malcolm E, Moss AH. Palliative care disincentives in CKD: Changing policy to improve CKD care. American Journal of Kidney Diseases. 2018;**71**(6):866. Available from: https://pmc.ncbi.nlm.nih.gov/articles/PMC5970958/

[22] Raja SN, Carr DB, Cohen M, Finnerup NB, Flor H, Gibson S, et al. The revised international association for the study of pain definition of pain: Concepts, challenges, and compromises. Pain. 2020;**161**(9):1976-1982. Available from: https://pubmed.ncbi.nlm.nih.gov/32694387/

[23] Ernecoff NC, Bell LF, Arnold RM, Shea CM, Switzer GE, Jhamb M, et al. Clinicians' perceptions of collaborative palliative care delivery in chronic kidney disease. Journal of Pain and Symptom Management. 2022;**64**(2):168-177.

Available from: https://pubmed.ncbi.nlm.nih.gov/35417752/

[24] Lanini I, Samoni S, Husain-Syed F, Fabbri S, Canzani F, Messeri A, et al. Palliative care for patients with kidney disease. Journal of Clinical Medicine. 2022;**11**(13):3923. Available from: https://pmc/articles/PMC9267754/

[25] Fiseha T, Osborne NJ. Burden of end-stage renal disease of undetermined etiology in Africa. Renal Replacement Therapy. 2023;**9**(1):1-10. DOI: 10.1186/s41100-023-00497-w

[26] Francis A, Abdul Hafidz MI, Ekrikpo UE, Chen T, Wijewickrama E, Tannor EK, et al. Barriers to accessing essential medicines for kidney disease in low- and lower middle-income countries|. Kidney International. 2022;**102**(5):969-973. Available from: https://pubmed.ncbi.nlm.nih.gov/36044940/

[27] Naicker S. Nephrology in Africa - challenges of practice in resource-limited environment. Clinical Nephrology. 2016;**86**(13):84-89. Available from: https://pubmed.ncbi.nlm.nih.gov/27469153/

[28] Arogundade FA, Barsoum RS. CKD prevention in sub-Saharan Africa: A call for governmental, nongovernmental, and community support. American Journal of Kidney Diseases. 2008;**51**(3):515-523. Available from: http://www.ajkd.org/article/S0272638607015995/fulltext

[29] Carney EF. The impact of chronic kidney disease on global health. Nature Reviews. Nephrology. 2020;**16**(5):251. Available from: https://www.researchgate.net/publication/339751744_The_impact_of_chronic_kidney_disease_on_global_health

[30] Yeates K, Ghosh S, Kilonzo K. Developing nephrology programs in very low-resource settings: Challenges in sustainability. Kidney International. Supplement. 2013;**3**(2):202-205

[31] Elrggal ME, Bek SG, Shendi AM, Tannor EK, Nlandu YM, Gaipov A. Disparities in access to kidney transplantation in developing countries. Transplantation. 2021;**105**(11):2325-2329. Available from: https://pubmed.ncbi.nlm.nih.gov/34709218/

[32] White SL, Chadban SJ, Jan S, Chapman JR, Cass A. How can we achieve global equity in provision of renal replacement therapy? Bulletin of the World Health Organization. 2008;**86**(3):229-237. Available from: https://pubmed.ncbi.nlm.nih.gov/18368211/

[33] Wong G, Bernier-Jean A, Rovin B, Ronco P. Time for action: Recognizing chronic kidney disease as a major noncommunicable disease driver of premature mortality. Kidney International. 2024;**105**(6):1144-1146. Available from: http://www.kidney-international.org/article/S0085253824002473/fulltext

[34] McKnight M, Dufatanye E, Rugamba G, Ntarindwa J, Igirineza G, Vos P, et al. Sun-223 implementation of a renal biopsy program in Rwanda: A feasibility study. Kidney International Reports. 2019;**4**(7):S251-S252. Available from: http://www.kireports.org/article/S246802491930823X/fulltext

[35] Ayodele OE, Alebiosu CO. Burden of chronic kidney disease: An international perspective. Advances in Chronic Kidney Disease. 2010;**17**(3):215-224. Available from: https://pubmed.ncbi.nlm.nih.gov/20439090/

[36] Marie Patrice H, Joiven N, Hermine F, Jean Yves B, Folefack François K, Enow GA. Factors associated

with late presentation of patients with chronic kidney disease in nephrology consultation in Cameroon-a descriptive cross-sectional study. Renal Failure. 2019;**41**(1):384-392. Available from: https://www.researchgate.net/publication/333224865_Factors_associated_with_late_presentation_of_patients_with_chronic_kidney_disease_in_nephrology_consultation_in_Cameroon-a_descriptive_cross-sectional_study

[37] Jha V, Rathi M. Natural medicines causing acute kidney injury. Seminars in Nephrology. 2008;**28**(4):416-428. Available from: https://pubmed.ncbi.nlm.nih.gov/18620964/

[38] Osman MA, Alrukhaimi M, Ashuntantang GE, Bellorin-Font E, Benghanem Gharbi M, Braam B, et al. Global nephrology workforce: Gaps and opportunities toward a sustainable kidney care system. Kidney International. Supplement. 2018;**8**(2):52-63. Available from: https://pubmed.ncbi.nlm.nih.gov/30675439/

[39] Metzger M, Abdel-Rahman EM, Boykin H, Song MK. A narrative review of management strategies for common symptoms in advanced CKD. Kidney International Reports. 2021;**6**(4):894. Available from: https://pmc.ncbi.nlm.nih.gov/articles/PMC8071652/

[40] Roy PJ, Weltman M, Dember LM, Liebschutz J, Jhamb M. Pain management in patients with chronic kidney disease and end-stage kidney disease. Current Opinion in Nephrology and Hypertension. 2020;**29**(6):671. Available from: https://pmc.ncbi.nlm.nih.gov/articles/PMC7753951/

[41] Parker Gregg L, Bossola M, Ostrosky-Frid M, Susan Hedayati S. Fatigue in CKD: Epidemiology, pathophysiology, and treatment. Clinical Journal of the American Society of Nephrology. 2021;**16**(9):1445. Available from: https://pmc.ncbi.nlm.nih.gov/articles/PMC8729574/

[42] Koncicki HM, Unruh M, Schell JO. Pain management in CKD: A guide for nephrology providers. American Journal of Kidney Diseases. 2017;**69**(3):451-460. Available from: http://www.ajkd.org/article/S0272638616305595/fulltext

[43] Lambourg E, Colvin L, Guthrie G, Walker H, Bell S. Analgesic use and associated adverse events in patients with chronic kidney disease: A systematic review and meta-analysis. British Journal of Anaesthesia. 2022;**128**(3):546-561. Available from: http://www.bjanaesthesia.org/article/S0007091221006401/fulltext

[44] Lipman ZM, Paramasivam V, Yosipovitch G, Germain MJ. Clinical management of chronic kidney disease-associated pruritus: Current treatment options and future approaches. Clinical Kidney Journal. 2021;**14**(Suppl. 3):i16. Available from: https://pmc.ncbi.nlm.nih.gov/articles/PMC8702820/

[45] Rigatto C, Collister D, Granger-Vallée A, Girard L, Hingwala J, Karaboyas A, et al. Pathways for diagnosing and treating ckd-associated pruritus: A narrative review. Canadian Journal of Kidney Health and Disease [Internet]. 1 Jan 2024;**11**:20543581241238808. DOI: 10.1177/20543581241238808. [cited 2024 Dec 3]; Available from: https://journals.sagepub.com/doi/10.1177/20543581241238808

[46] Goh ZS, Griva K. Anxiety and depression in patients with end-stage renal disease: Impact and management challenges—A narrative review. International Journal of Nephrology and Renovascular Disease. 2018;**11**:93.

Available from: https://pmc.ncbi.nlm.nih.gov/articles/PMC5856029/

[47] Draganović S, Kurulmaz B. Depression and anxiety levels among chronic kidney patients. Epiphany. 2019;**11**(1):31

[48] Roy SR, Ishrar SMG, Caleerappa R, Reddy VB, Chenna N, Chapiri DL, et al. Impact of stress, anxiety, and depression on chronic kidney disease and its effects on quality of life. Global Journal of Medical Pharmaceutical and Biomedical Update [Internet]. 16 May 2024;**19**:3.10.25259/GJMPBU_108_2023. [cited 2024 Dec 4]; DOI: 10.25259/GJMPBU. Available from: https://gjmpbu.org/impact-of-stress-anxiety-and-depression-on-chronic-kidney-disease-and-its-effects-on-quality-of-life/

[49] Tu CY, Chou YH, Lin YH, Huang WL. Sleep and emotional disturbance in patients with non-dialysis chronic kidney disease. Journal of the Formosan Medical Association. 2019;**118**(6):986-994. Available from: https://pubmed.ncbi.nlm.nih.gov/30416021/

[50] Adejumo OA, Iyawe IO, Akinbodewa AA, Abolarin OS, Alli EO. Burden, psychological well-being and quality of life of caregivers of end stage renal disease patients. Ghana Medical Journal. 2019;**53**(3):190-196

[51] Senanayake S, Gunawardena N, Palihawadana P, Suraweera C, Karunarathna R, Kumara P. Depression and psychological distress in patients with chronic renal failure: Prevalence and associated factors in a rural district in Sri Lanka. Journal of Psychosomatic Research. 2018;**112**:25-31. Available from: https://pubmed.ncbi.nlm.nih.gov/30097132/

[52] Hettiarachchi R, Abeysena C. Association of poor social support and financial insecurity with psychological distress of chronic kidney disease patients attending national nephrology unit in Sri Lanka. International Journal of Nephrology [Internet]. 2018;**2018**:5678781. DOI: 10.1155/2018/5678781. [cited 2024 Dec 4]; Available from: https://pubmed.ncbi.nlm.nih.gov/29888004/

[53] Nair D. Measuring and modifying psychological distress in CKD: New insights and next steps. Kidney Medicine. 2019;**1**(4):147. Available from: https://pmc.ncbi.nlm.nih.gov/articles/PMC7380378/

[54] Francis A, Harhay MN, Ong ACM, Tummalapalli SL, Ortiz A, Fogo AB, et al. Chronic kidney disease and the global public health agenda: An international consensus. Nature Reviews. Nephrology. 2024;**20**(7):473-485. Available from: https://www.nature.com/articles/s41581-024-00820-6

[55] Stephenson GK. ISN–Global kidney health atlas, 3rd ed: A report by the international society of nephrology: An assessment of global kidney health care status focusing on capacity, availability, accessibility, affordability and outcomes of kidney disease. International Society of Nephrology. 2023:19-28. Available from: http://www.theisn.org/global-atlas; www.theisn.org/global-atlas

[56] Obrador GT, Rubilar X, Agazzi E, Estefan J. The challenge of providing renal replacement therapy in developing countries: The Latin American perspective. American Journal of Kidney Diseases. 2016;**67**(3):499-506. Available from: https://pubmed.ncbi.nlm.nih.gov/26709109/

[57] Earnshaw VA, Quinn DM. The impact of stigma in healthcare on people living with chronic illnesses. Journal of Health Psychology. 2011;**17**(2):157.

Available from: https://pmc.ncbi.nlm.nih.gov/articles/PMC8919040/

[58] Luyckx VA, Tonelli M, Stanifer JW. The global burden of kidney disease and the sustainable development goals. Bulletin of the World Health Organization. 2018;**96**(6):414. Available from: https://pmc.ncbi.nlm.nih.gov/articles/PMC5996218/

[59] Davison SN. Integrating palliative care for patients with advanced chronic kidney disease: Recent advances, remaining challenges. Journal of Palliative Care. Spring; 2011;**27**(1):53-61

[60] Patel V, Chowdhary N, Rahman A, Verdeli H. Improving access to psychological treatments: Lessons from developing countries. Behaviour Research and Therapy. 2011;**49**(9):523-528. Available from: https://pubmed.ncbi.nlm.nih.gov/21788012/

[61] Knaul FM, Farmer PE, Krakauer EL, De Lima L, Bhadelia A, Jiang Kwete X, et al. Alleviating the access abyss in palliative care and pain relief—An imperative of universal health coverage: The lancet commission report. Lancet. 2018;**391**(10128):1391-1454. Available from: http://www.thelancet.com/article/S0140673617325138/fulltext

[62] Koenig HG. Religion, spirituality, and health: The research and clinical implications. ISRN Psychiatry. 2012;**2012**:278730. Available from: https://pmc.ncbi.nlm.nih.gov/articles/PMC3671693/

[63] Yodchai K, Dunning T, Savage S, Hutchinson AM. The role of religion and spirituality in coping with kidney disease and haemodialysis in Thailand. Scandinavian Journal of Caring Sciences. 2017;**31**(2):359-367. Available from: https://pubmed.ncbi.nlm.nih.gov/27327262/

[64] Philips PL, Lazenby M. The emotional and spiritual well-being of hospice patients in Botswana and sources of distress for their caregivers. Journal of Palliative Medicine. 2013;**16**(11):1438-1445. Available from: https://www.researchgate.net/publication/257299791_The_Emotional_and_Spiritual_Well-Being_of_Hospice_Patients_in_Botswana_and_Sources_of_Distress_for_Their_Caregivers

[65] Egan R, Wood S, Macleod R, Walker R. Spirituality in renal supportive care: A thematic review. Healthcare. 2015;**3**(4):1174-1193. Available from: https://www.mdpi.com/2227-9032/3/4/1174/htm

[66] Kagawa-Singer M, Blackhall LJ. Negotiating cross-cultural issues at the end of life: "You got to go where he lives". JAMA. 2001;**286**(23):2993-3001. Available from: https://pubmed.ncbi.nlm.nih.gov/11743841/

[67] Basirika D, Merriman A, Gumoyesige N, Namisango E, Matthews E, Guma S. Insights into advance care planning in Africa. Zeitschrift für Evidenz, Fortbildung und Qualität im Gesundheitswesen. 2023;**180**:16-20

[68] Deodhar J, Nagaraju SP, Kirpalani AL, Nayak AM, Deodhar J, Nagaraju SP, et al. Shared decision-making, advance care planning for chronic kidney disease patients. Indian Journal of Palliative Care. 2021;**27**(Suppl. 1):S33-S36. Available from: https://jpalliativecare.com/shared-decision-making-advance-care-planning-for-chronic-kidney-disease-patients/

[69] Raghavan D, Holley JL. Conservative care of the elderly CKD patient: A practical guide. Advances in Chronic Kidney Disease. Jan 2016;**23**(1):51-56. DOI: 10.1053/j.ackd.2015.08.003. [cited 2024 Feb 21]

[70] Frandsen CE, Dieperink H, Trettin B, Agerskov H. Advance care planning to patients with chronic kidney disease and their families: An intervention development study. Journal of Clinical Nursing. 2023;**32**(23-24):8104-8115. Available from: https://pubmed.ncbi.nlm.nih.gov/37743635/

[71] O'Halloran P, Noble H, Norwood K, Maxwell P, Shields J, Fogarty D, et al. Advance care planning with patients who have end-stage kidney disease: A systematic realist review. Journal of Pain and Symptom Management. 2018;**56**(5):795. Available from: https://pmc.ncbi.nlm.nih.gov/articles/PMC6203056/

[72] Guma S, Namisango E, Ddungu H. Advance care planning and palliative care for patients with advanced cancer in Uganda. Zeitschrift für Evidenz, Fortbildung und Qualität im Gesundheitswesen. 2023;**180**:29-35. Available from: https://pubmed.ncbi.nlm.nih.gov/37550121/

[73] Bagasha P, Namukwaya E, Leng M, Kalyesubula R, Mutebi E, Naitala R, et al. Comparison of the health-related quality of life of end stage kidney disease patients on hemodialysis and non-hemodialysis management in Uganda. BMC Palliative Care. 2021;**20**(1):1-13. Available from: https://bmcpalliatcare.biomedcentral.com/articles/10.1186/s12904-021-00743-0

[74] Russon L, Mooney A. Palliative and end-of-life care in advanced renal failure. Clinical Medicine (Northfield IL). 2010;**10**(3):279. Available from: https://pmc.ncbi.nlm.nih.gov/articles/PMC5873558/

[75] Prabhu R, Salins N, Bharathi B, Abraham G. End of life care in end-stage kidney disease. Indian Journal of Palliative Care. 2021;**27**(5):S37-S42. Available from: https://www.researchgate.net/publication/351958302_End_of_Life_Care_in_End-Stage_Kidney_Disease

[76] Vélez-López A, Carmona-Torres JM, López-González Á, Laredo-Aguilera JA, Callado-Pérez D, Rabanales-Sotos J. Community-based interventions in people with palliative care needs: An integrative review of studies from 2017 to 2022. Healthcare. 2024;**12**(15):1477. Available from: https://pmc.ncbi.nlm.nih.gov/articles/PMC11311615/

[77] Surendran P, Venugopal V, Dongre A, Paninjukunnath R. Perceived challenges faced by family caregivers of chronic kidney disease patients and suggested solutions: A qualitative study. International Journal of Medical Science and Public Health [Internet]. 2018;**7**(6):487-492. DOI: 10.5455/ijmsph.2018.0307819032018. [cited 2024 Dec 7]. Available from: https://www.researchgate.net/publication/324097616_Perceived_challenges_faced_by_family_caregivers_of_chronic_kidney_disease_patients_and_suggested_solutions_A_qualitative_study

[78] Wee LX, Tan PST, Chen HC. Experiences and needs of families caring for children and adolescents with chronic kidney disease: A meta-synthesis. Journal of Pediatric Nursing. 2022;**63**:52-63. Available from: https://pubmed.ncbi.nlm.nih.gov/35007849/

[79] Vieira IF d O, Paiva EM d C, SMCL F. Burden and social support in caregivers of people with kidney disease: A systematic integrative review. Brazilian Journal of Health Review. 2023;**6**(2):5620-5638. Available from: https://ojs.brazilianjournals.com.br/ojs/index.php/BJHR/article/view/58141

[80] Ania-González N, Martín-Martín J, Amezqueta-Goñi P,

Vázquez-Calatayud M. The needs of families who care for individuals with kidney failure on comprehensive conservative care: A qualitative systematic review. Journal of Renal Care. 2022;**48**(4):230. Available from: https://pmc.ncbi.nlm.nih.gov/articles/PMC9790615/

[81] Manera KE, Gutman T, Finkelstein F, Tong A. Family and caregiver support. In: Evidence-Based Nephrology [Internet]. 2nd ed. Vol. 2. 12 Jan Wiley; 2022:584-9. DOI: 10.1002/9781119105954. [cited 2024 Dec 7]; Available from: https://onlinelibrary.wiley.com/doi/full/10.1002/9781119105954.ch78

[82] Abu-Odah H, Molassiotis A, Liu J. Challenges on the provision of palliative care for patients with cancer in low- and middle-income countries: a systematic review of reviews. BMC Palliative Care [Internet]. 22 Apr 2020;**19**(1):55. DOI: 10.1186/s12904-020-00558-5. [cited 2024 Nov 26]

[83] Sturgill D, Bear A. Unique palliative care needs of patients with advanced chronic kidney disease – The scope of the problem and several solutions. Clinical Medicine (Northfield IL). 2019;**19**(1):26-29. Available from: https://www.rcpjournals.org/content/clinmedicine/19/1/26

[84] Gelfand SL, Schell J, Eneanya ND. Palliative care in nephrology: The work and the workforce. Advances in Chronic Kidney Disease. 2020;**27**(4):350-355.e1. Available from: https://www.researchgate.net/publication/346084487_Palliative_Care_in_Nephrology_The_Work_and_the_Workforce

[85] Swanepoel CR, McCulloch MI, Abraham G, Donner JA, Alrukhaimi MN, Blake PG, et al. Challenges for sustainable end-stage kidney disease care in low-middle-income countries: The problem of the workforce. Kidney International. Supplement. 2020;**10**(1):e49. Available from: https://pmc.ncbi.nlm.nih.gov/articles/PMC7031680/

[86] Brock G, Blake M. What should be done to address losses associated with "medical brain drain"? Journal of Medical Ethics. 2017;**43**(8):558-559. Available from: https://www.researchgate.net/publication/301539399_What_should_be_done_to_address_losses_associated_with_'medical_brain_drain'

[87] Oladeji BD, Gureje O. Brain drain: A challenge to global mental health. BJPsych International. 2016;**13**(3):61-63. Available from: https://pubmed.ncbi.nlm.nih.gov/29093905/

[88] Hannon B, Zimmermann C, Knaul FM, Powell RA, Mwangi-Powell FN, Rodin G. Provision of palliative Care in low- and Middle-Income Countries: Overcoming obstacles for effective treatment delivery. Journal of Clinical Oncology. 2016;**34**(1):62-68. DOI: 10.1200/JCO.2015.62.1615

[89] Reid E, Ghoshal A, Khalil A, Jiang J, Normand C, Brackett A, et al. Out-of-pocket costs near end of life in low- and middle-income countries: A systematic review. PLOS Global Public Health. 2022;**2**(1):e0000005. Available from: https://pmc.ncbi.nlm.nih.gov/articles/PMC10022295/

[90] Dodd R, Palagyi A, Guild L, Jha V, Jan S. The impact of out-of-pocket costs on treatment commencement and adherence in chronic kidney disease: A systematic review. Health Policy and Planning. 2018;**33**(9):1047-1054. Available from: https://pubmed.ncbi.nlm.nih.gov/30247548/

[91] Qarni B, Osman MA, Levin A, Feehally J, Harris D, Jindal K, et al. Kidney

care in low- and middle-income countries. Clinical Nephrology. 2020;**93**(1):S21-S30. Available from: https://pubmed.ncbi.nlm.nih.gov/31397271/

[92] Okolo CA, Olorunsogo T, Babawarun O. Cultural variability in pain perception: A review of cross-cultural studies. International Journal of Scientific Research. 2024;**11**(1):2550-2556

[93] Journal O, Ghali HH. Cultural challenges in implementing palliative care services in Iraq. Palliative Medicine and Hospice Care Open Journal. Special edition 1. 2017. DOI: 10.17140/PMHCOJ-SE-1-105. [cited 2024 Feb 18]

[94] Richardson P. Spirituality, religion and palliative care. Annals of Palliative Medicine. Jul 2016;**3**(3):150-159. DOI: 10.3978/j.issn.2224-5820.2014.07.05

[95] Bloomer MJ, Poon P, Runacres F, Hutchinson AM. Facilitating family needs and support at the end of life in hospital: A descriptive study. Palliative Medicine. 30 Dec 2021;**36**(3):549-554. DOI: 10.1177/02692163211066431. [cited 2023 Apr 20] Epub 2021 Dec 30. Available from: https://journals.sagepub.com/doi/full/10.1177/02692163211066431

[96] Mokgobi MG. Understanding traditional African healing. African Journal for Physical Activity and Health Sciences. 2014;**20**(Suppl. 2):24-34. Available from: http://www.ncbi.nlm.nih.gov/pubmed/26594664%0Ahttp://www.pubmedcentral.nih.gov/articlerender.fcgi?artid=PMC4651463

[97] Cherny NI. Stigma associated with "palliative care". Cancer. 2009;**115**(9):1808-1812. Available from: https://www.researchgate.net/publication/24033021_Stigma_Associated_With_Palliative_Care_Getting_Around_It_or_Getting_Over_It

[98] Logie DE. An evaluation of a public health advocacy strategy to enhance palliative care provision in Zambia. BMJ Supportive & Palliative Care. 2012;**2**(3):264-269. Available from: https://pubmed.ncbi.nlm.nih.gov/24654199/

[99] Canning D, Rosenberg JP, Yates P. Therapeutic relationships in specialist palliative care nursing practice. International Journal of Palliative Nursing. 2007;**13**(5):222-229. Available from: https://www.researchgate.net/publication/6260337_Theraputic_relationships_in_specialist_palliative_care_nursing_practice

[100] Salikhanov I, Katapodi MC, Kunirova G, Crape BL. Improving palliative care outcomes in remote and rural areas of LMICs through family caregivers: Lessons from Kazakhstan. Frontiers in Public Health. 2023;**11**:1186107. Available from: https://pmc.ncbi.nlm.nih.gov/articles/PMC10434554/

[101] Gordon B, Mason B, SLH S. Leveraging telehealth for delivery of palliative care to remote communities: A rapid review. Journal of Palliative Care. 2021;**37**(2):213. Available from: https://pmc.ncbi.nlm.nih.gov/articles/PMC9286776/

[102] van Heerden EM, Jenkins LS. The role of community health workers in palliative care in a rural subdistrict in South Africa. African Journal of Primary Health & Family Medicine. 2022;**14**(1):3657. Available from: https://pmc.ncbi.nlm.nih.gov/articles/PMC9724038/

Chapter 4

Perspective Chapter: Rekindling the Vision for Palliative and End-of-Life Care for Future Practices

Erna Haraldsdottir

Abstract

This chapter will focus on the original philosophy of palliative care as developed by Dame Cicely Saunders. Attention will be paid to the development of palliative care and the challenges to remain close to the original vision as practice develops further within a traditional medical environment. The overall purpose and focus of the chapter are for the reader to engage with the inherent holistic and person-centered approach of palliative and end-of-life care as developed by Cicely Saunders and to gain an understanding and insight into how to maintain her vision as an essential element of care within modern palliative and end-of-life care.

Keywords: palliative care, end-of-life care, developing practice, holistic care, philosophy of palliative care

1. Introduction

This chapter will focus on the original philosophy of palliative care as developed by Dame Cicely Saunders. Light is shed on the development of palliative care and the challenges to remain close to the original vision as palliative care develops and expands in reach and scope. A critical understanding of the medicalization of palliative and end-of-life care is provided with insights into the limitations of the traditional biomedical model for organizing and subculturing palliative and end-of-life care. I will show the unique contribution nursing brings to palliative and end-of-life care. In recognizing the alignment of Cicely Saunders' original philosophy and principles of palliative care with the underpinning theories, knowledge and skills of the nursing profession, I will argue how nursing leadership is vital as palliative care develops in reach and scope.

2. The original vision of palliative and end-of-life care

> *"You matter because you are you and you matter to the end of your life. We will do all we can not only to help you to die peacefully, but also to live until you die."*

These words of Dame Cicely Saunders, the founder of the hospice movement, are echoed in many current strategic documents and ambitions for palliative care end-of-life care services [1]. The words encapsulate Saunders' vision for a transformation of care for those who were dying and her request for a cultural shift in the attitudes toward death and dying within health care organizations and amongst health care professionals in the late 1950s and early 1960s [2].

Saunders developed her vision within the context of a health care system where death was seen as a failure and there was a lack of knowledge and skills to meet the needs of dying people in the ways they needed care. To meet this need, Saunders developed and implemented an innovative approach based on the philosophy and principles of an open awareness of death [3]. Saunders was educated as a nurse, social worker and medical doctor and she drew on her knowledge and skills from all these disciplines when developing her approach [4]. Through her sophisticated and reflective writings, based on her practice and observations, she established a philosophy and principles of care that still underpin the foundation of modern palliative and end-of-life care [4]. In the early 1970s, her approach was named "palliative care" by the Canadian surgeon Balfour Mount who was influenced by Saunders' approach and brought it to North America [5]. The World Health Organization has identified palliative care as an approach that improves the quality of life of patients—adults and children—and their families who are facing problems associated with life-threatening illnesses. It prevents and relieves suffering through the early identification, impeccable assessment and treatment of pain and other problems, whether physical, psychosocial or spiritual [6].

Saunders recognized, when developing her approach into practice in the 1960s, that her ideas were too radical to be accepted within the established culture of health care with its strong curative intent. Death was seen as a failure and health care staff both feared death and felt there was nothing they could do for dying people [2]. Hence, most people were left to die in hospitals in isolation and in loneliness and this was named as social death by the social scientist David Sudnow in 1967 [7]. Saunders developed the first modern hospice in South London, St Christopher's Hospice in 1967 and this was an organization outside the parameters of the British national health care system. The Hospice was a voluntary organization based on charitable funding with the core focus of looking after dying people with incurable cancer. The story of the opening of the hospice has a romantic element to it whereby Saunders developed a strong bond with one of her patients, David Tasma. He was dying in a busy hospital surgical ward in 1959. Saunders cared for him and discussed her new and innovative ideas for the care of the dying with him. David donated money after his death to Saunders toward a window in her "home" (referring to the organization she wanted to establish) [4].

3. Development of palliative and end-of-life care

The palliative care approach has developed globally and is integrated, at least at some levels, into most health care systems across the world with an identified need for further development in low- and middle-income countries [8]. Much has been achieved with the development of palliative and end-of-life care across the world, and this should be celebrated. However, as palliative and end-of-life care has developed and been integrated into established health care systems, it is important to consider and pay attention to the challenges this poses to the creative and innovative vision of

Cicely Saunders. It has been highlighted that during this integration process, palliative and end-of-life care has become medicalized [9]. Established health care systems are underpinned by the biomedical model of illness that has dominated health care for the past century [10]. With its biologically dependent perspective, there is a hierarchy of knowledge and perspective as being disease-oriented, whereby health is seen as the removal and absence of disease [10]. Palliative and end-of-life care has become integrated into the administrative machine of the traditional health care system influenced heavily by the medical bioscience perspective whereby processes to regulate and stabilize the system are set by this perspective [11].

The Hospice movement started as a pioneering movement, led by Saunders who by her own agency and personal interest promoted a new values orientation within health care. Death should not be seen as a failure but at times the unavoidable consequences of an illness. In responding to the needs of the dying, health professionals needed to provide care in a new and creative way for people who were not able to be cured. Whilst Saunders' original approach has remained the core focus of palliative and end-of-life care as it develops into health care practice across the world, it can be argued that her original vision has been diluted by the medical model in this development. The hierarchy of medical knowledge and perspective has led to a focus on symptom management based on biomedical science and the development of interventions to remove symptoms based on the medical model. The more creative and humanistic approach to care as promoted by Saunders has gained less attention, funding and resources. This focus and priority can be explained by the fact that with the integration into the main health care system, palliative care has developed from an innovative grassroots movement into a structure, rules and organization whereby the core function is based on the traditional biomedical model.

The early hospice movement was innovative in its organization and care as there were no rules to follow and no established authorities or organizations to set standards. Within this environment, a new culture of care was established through an integrated system of belief, behavior and knowledge. Common values and purpose were developed that attracted individuals who identified with these and wanted to work within such a setting. In developing this culture, Saunders was a charismatic leader with commitment, creativity and disruption who created new structures and a system for care [4].

Saunders said that she took care of the dying out of the British national health care system to bring it back into the system [11, 12]. With this transition, palliative and end-of-life care practice was routinized and has become subject to bureaucracy and governance of a medical-orientated system [11].

The positive impact of palliative care and end-of-life care becoming integrated into the main health care systems is widely recognized. However, with this development, the medicalization of Saunders' original vision has been dominant. This has led to less of an emphasis on practice based on the aspects of Saunders' vision being underpinned by concepts such as personhood, meaning and personal growth. When developing her pioneering approach, these were the core elements of care, alongside the focus on symptoms and symptom management, based on the medical model, in equal measure. Saunders understood the limitation of medical knowledge alone when developing her model of care. She advocated for a humanistic orientation of care, whereby the hierarchy of medicine was challenged, and an emphasis was put on teamwork and ensuring that the person who was ill and his/her family were at the center of care [4]. Saunders replaced the passive approach and the notion that there was nothing health care professionals could do for those who were dying, based on the medical model, with her new model of active care. This new and innovative approach was based on innovative and creative ways of continuing caring up to the end of life and beyond for the family [4].

To demonstrate the understanding and need for her approach, Saunders introduced the concept of "total pain." This concept remains a key concept in modern palliative care and in developing this concept, Saunders recognized the interdependency of mind, soul and body. She identified that for dying people, there was a type of suffering that manifested itself in the feeling of "everything is wrong" [13]. Saunders understood the limitation of the medical model to relieve this type of suffering, and she developed a more humanistic and creative approach to this, namely "being with" [14]. Michael Kearney further expounded upon Saunders' work and highlighted the difference between the model of total pain and the medical model of pain. He demonstrated that interventions based on the traditional medical model are not able to alleviate the type of pain Saunders described as total pain by differentiating between pain of a biological nature with pain of an existential nature [13]. Kearney and Saunders both brought to light how people facing incurable illnesses and imminent death may experience pain and suffering caused by disruption to personhood and existence, causing existential anxiety and suffering. The pain experienced may have little to do with disease or physical symptoms of a disease but is embedded deeply within the person. This pain may aggravate physical pain but the causes of this type of pain are of a different nature and caused by a sense of loss and an overwhelming emotion that life is ending [13, 15].

4. Palliative care nursing

I have demonstrated in this chapter how the medicalization and routinization of Saunders' original vision, principles and philosophy with the biomedical model of health care took hold of palliative and end-of-life care [16]. I will now turn to focus on the consequences of this for nursing and the importance of the voice of nursing to be clearly heard in the development of palliative and end-of-life care [17–19].

The creative and care aspect of Saunders' principles and philosophy aligns very well with the theories and models that underpin nursing practice such as the focus on relationship-centered care, the essence of nursing as a connection to the patient experience and humanistic care [19, 20]. Moran et al. provide important evidence of the role and contribution of the nurse in caring for people with palliative care and their families. Within their thematic analysis, the multiple and complex roles of the nurse and nursing are identified through eight domains—person-centered care, positive interpersonal behaviors, medical/nursing and technical competency, clinical leadership and governance, management of the environment, promotion of safety and evidence-based practice [20].

Nurses are the largest regulated health care professional workforce providing palliative care across a range of clinical settings [19]. Nurses in palliative care engage in a wide range of roles and responsibilities in caring for people with palliative care needs and their families and the caring and artistic role of nurses is fundamental to palliative and end-of-life care [20]. Whilst nursing aligns so strongly with the underpinning philosophy of palliative care, as palliative and end-of-life care has been integrated into the mainstream health care system, there has been a lack of visibility of the nursing contribution to palliative care and their essential role. Palliative care nursing has been subsumed as palliative care medicine has developed, with the voice of nursing being silenced, and the artistic element of nursing being diluted [19, 20]. The nursing role has developed into being an assistance role rather than a leading role within the care of those needing palliative and end-of-life care [20]. However, nursing values strongly reflect the values that shaped the principles and philosophies of palliative care as developed by Saunders such as care, compassion, courage and fostering growth. Nursing in its essence has its focus on every person as unique in their story and this profoundly impacts the way care needs are being assessed and delivered to patients and their families when supporting living through the final stage of life. The care plan is set up and delivered by a responsive and flexible approach whereby the whole care team may intervene effectively in different areas of suffering and need. This approach considers and appreciates the entirety of the ill person, the whole family and their community. Nursing care and relationships form the pillar of the care plan whereby the caring team brings kindness and compassion, an authentic presence, and understands how transformation and personal growth can be fostered through relationships [21].

5. Development of models of palliative and end-of-life care

The negative impact of the medicalization of palliative care and end-of-life care has been recognized [9, 16] and new models of palliative care have been emerging over the last decades. These models of care are much more appreciative of the contribution of disciplines other than medicine such as Dignity-Conserving Care [22]. Others emphasize the need to go beyond the clinical perspective and include communities in palliative and end-of-life care [23]. Within these new care models, there is much more of an emphasis on the non-medical aspects of care with the scope for more creative and humanistic care, as emphasized by Saunders.

Recent developments, and perhaps the most influential global discussion in modern health and social care, revolve around the person-centered model of care. This model of care has been highly influential and person-centered care and is promoted in many policies and strategies of health care [24]. The core essence of the person-centered model of care is to shift the focus from a medically dominated and disease-orientated framework toward one that is relationship-focused and holistic [25]. This approach to health care encourages valuing people for who they are as individuals rather than focusing on diagnostic categories, whilst also facilitating positive relationships through honest information sharing and open communication [26].

The person-centered framework by McCormack and McCance was developed to operationalize person-centeredness in health care practice with its theoretical underpinning based on humanistic care [27]. The framework consists of person-centered processes that focus on ways of engaging that are necessary to create connections between people, which include working with the person's beliefs and values and engaging authentically, being sympathetic present, sharing decision-making and working holistically [27]. This focus on engagement and the broader health care needs assessment and care is much less based on diagnostic categories than the medical model and aligns very well with Saunders' model of palliative and end-of-life care. Furthermore, within the person-centered framework, it is recognized that there is an interlinking of disease and its symptoms with experience, gender, age and social circumstances which brings an interplay of factors that needs to be assessed through a lens that is person-centered and goes beyond the traditional medical assessment [28]. Within person-centered care, there is an emphasis on personhood and the desire to keep the person in the center of decision-making, hence challenging the biomedical model with its focus on medical labels and system efficacy that may not have the person at the heart of its care [27]. Personhood refers to an innate sense of ourselves as human beings with feelings, emotions, thoughts and desires, it is an inner feeling that guides and gives a sense of "what really matters" [29]. The person-centered model of care aligns very well with Saunders' unwavering focus on what matters to the individual and those close to this individual. Through this lens, both person-centered care and the palliative care approach, as developed by Saunders, reflect the ideals of humanistic caring. Whereby there is a moral component, and practice has at its basis a therapeutic intent, which is translated through relationships that are built on effective interpersonal processes [27]. Attention is paid to health care needs with a holistic perspective that aims to support well-being within each situation. This reflects a much broader notion of health than the medical model and reflects a perspective on health care where a focus is on living a positive life which embraces all dimensions of our being [30].

McCormack and McCance emphasize that operationalizing the person-centered framework in practice requires a cultural shift due to the medicalization of health care [31]. Culture embraces a social context that influences the way people behave and talk and the social norms that are accepted and expected. Hence, transforming culture and shifting how things are done on a practice level requires a fundamental change in mindset, language and behavior [30]. Palliative care needs to be transformed with a cultural shift to challenge the old traditional biomedical model being the dominating perspective when structuring and organizing care that meets the needs of people with long-term conditions and who are facing imminent death. This is increasingly important as palliative and end-of-life care is being recognized as an effective model of care, not only for people with cancer but also for other long-term conditions and early in the disease trajectory [32]. As the demand increases, palliative and end-of-life care needs to develop in reach and scope. It is vital for this development that the hierarchy of knowledge and perspective through the medical model is challenged. The contribution of other health care professionals such as nurses needs to be recognized as having the same value as medicine. The structure and organization of care need to focus on assessing the needs for care, where the needs for medical care are not prioritized, and seen as the most important and fundamental for meeting the holistic needs of people with palliative and end-of-life care needs and their families. This requires a cultural shift in language and behaviors challenging the embedded and traditional medical perspective. Further to this, the value of care provided by skilled social care needs to be seen in the right light. This is at times the core and main care provision needed to meet the holistic needs of people with incurable diseases and who are dying.

There is a tendency to focus on specialist and general palliative care when describing how palliative care needs to expand in scope and reach for everyone who can benefit from this approach having access. Interestingly, this classification and way of structuring and organizing care are based on the medical perspective. General palliative care is often seen as being delivered by all health care staff whereby specialist palliative care is provided by health care professionals with specialist knowledge. Within these differences in care delivery and need, the medical perspective based on biomedical science is evident. The difference is based on symptom management where it is seen that less complex symptoms can be managed by generalist health care providers, whereas more complex symptoms need specialist input. This overshadows the special knowledge and skills needed to meet the humanistic and creative caring approach based on interpersonal skills. This dual perspective overly focuses on symptoms and

DOI: http://dx.doi.org/10.5772/intechopen.1008971

symptom management as the essence of palliative care. Within this perspective, there is a hierarchy of care needs based on the medical model. This means that the specialist input needed for creative and humanistic care remains hidden and unspoken.

6. Developing future models for palliative and end-of-life care

Many people with incurable illnesses who are facing death do not need input from the medical profession. The same would apply to their family. Their needs are based on holistic needs whereby nursing care with its focus on humanity and creative approaches to care is needed. For many people wishing to be cared for and die at home, this is their core need, and the organization and structure of care need to be focused on this. Evidence shows that when structure and organization of care are based on this need and not overshadowed by the medical models such as a new nursing-led hospice-at-home model, this can avoid unnecessary admissions to inpatient wards [33]. Rather than focusing on organizing care based on generalist or specialist input, there is a need for a model of care with a comprehensive approach to care. This model of care allows for an assessment where the needs of people are not assessed through the lens of the medical model but through a much broader and holistic assessment of the need for care. The care may be led by a nurse or a skilled palliative social carer with a coordinated approach where other professionals, either generalist health care providers or specialist palliative care professionals, contribute to the care as needed.

For this model of care to be operationalized in a systematic way across health care systems, there needs to be a cultural shift from the way medicalization is currently dominating the structure and organization of care. This cultural change may take the same courage and disruption as demonstrated by Saunders' charismatic leadership in the 1960s as new ways of thinking and practicing need to be allowed to surface. It is worth noting that Saunders felt she needed to take palliative and end-of-life care out of the British national system to have the freedom to develop her approach. Within her new organization, St Christiopher's Hospice, she was able to create a new culture allowing for innovative approaches to be developed. However, the cultural shift needed now must happen within the health care system to continue to build on the current impact and success. In the United Kingdom, innovative approaches and models of care are happening in pockets of good practice in local areas but are often initiated by hospices and provided within the boundaries of the community of a hospice rather than being integrated into the main health care system in a consistent and integrated way. This needs to change and the integration of a holistic model needs to be integrated and expanded on through systematic and cultural change. It is vital for palliative and end-of-life care to be reoriented and organized in a truly holistic way to meet the demand for palliative care as it develops in its reach and scope.

7. Nurse-led palliative and end-of-life care

Nursing leadership and the voice of nursing are fundamental for the shift to the systematic and consistent delivery of a holistic model of palliative and end-of-life care. As highlighted earlier in this chapter, based on the theoretical underpinning and knowledge and skills of the nursing profession, nurses are in a key position to demonstrate leadership and challenge the medical dominance of the organization and structure of palliative care as it develops. To guide and support this shift, the Lantern model, a contemporary model of nursing and end-of-life care, was developed by two palliative care nurses in the UK [34]. The Lantern model builds on the Person-Centered Practice framework developed by McCormack and McCance [27]. The core aim of the model is to support nurse leadership and enable nurses to recognize and articulate the value the profession brings to palliative and end-of-life care through leadership and change [34]. The model offers visibility and a language to describe the unique contribution of nursing to palliative and end-of-life care as described by Saunders earlier in this chapter.

As highlighted earlier, within modern health care, the creative and humanistic aspect of care often remains hidden and unrecognized within a health care structure dominated by a discourse influenced by the medical model. This causes important interventions based on nursing care to have less priority. For example, the research highlighted how "being with," as developed by Saunders and highlighted by the person-centered framework as being present, was absent from the nursing practice in the hospice where the research took place. This was due to the way care was prioritized and provided through a structure and a system that did not value this type of engagement [14]. The overfocus of the medical model within the system and organization of care can also lead to misjudgment about what constitutes core health care priority. From the broader perspective, a need is seen as a specific indicator for needing health care intervention to control a problem which is negatively affecting well-being from a holistic perspective [35]. Through the narrow lens of the medical model overshadowing the broader perspective, there is a danger of bias whereby the assessment of needs is clouded by the medical lens. For example, a study into who is admitted, and why, to an inpatient ward from the community demonstrated how emotional safety and generally feeling safe was underestimated. This need was not seen as a core need for people wishing to be cared for and die at home due to the way the care was organized and structured. This led to people being admitted to inpatient hospices where the need for admission was masked by medical symptoms for admission to meet the right criteria. However, had the feeling of need for emotional safety at home been recognized as a core need and care organized and structured around this, the person would not have needed to be admitted [33].

The overmedicalization of palliative care can lead to misjudgment as to what health care service is needed for people needing palliative and end-of-life care. Not recognizing the real need can be costly and lead to the delivery of "right care at the right place" being compromised [36]. There is an urgent need for a comprehensive model of care to be integrated systematically into health care delivery whereby the holistic and person-centered vision of Saunders is being recognized in the way care is organized, structured and delivered.

8. Conclusion

In this chapter, I have highlighted the unique contribution of nursing to palliative and end-of-life care and how the value and care orientation of nursing practice toward humanist care based on interpersonal skills has been overshadowed by the medical model. Further to this, I have highlighted how as palliative care develops with further integration into the modern health care system, it is vital for cultural change to happen whereby the humanistic and creative care processes are recognized as fundamental elements of the model of care. For this cultural shift to happen, language,

DOI: http://dx.doi.org/10.5772/intechopen.1008971

behavior and practices based on the dominance of the medical perspective need to be challenged. Nurses need a stronger voice and clear language to lead this change effectively. A holistic model of care needs to underpin all palliative and end-of-life care practices whereby emphasis is on meeting a specific need for palliative and end-of-life care that may or may not be of a medical nature. This model of care puts less emphasis on the distinction between generalist and specialist palliative care services and more on specialist skills and knowledge provided by a variety of health care professionals and expert social careers. Nurses are in a primary position to lead such care.

Conflict of interest

The authors declare no conflict of interest.

Author details

Erna Haraldsdottir
Queen Margaret University, Edinburgh, Scotland

*Address all correspondence to: eharaldsdottir@qmu.ac.uk

References

[1] You Matter Because You are You An Action Plan for Better Palliative Care Cicely Saunders International [Internet]. 2021. Available from: https://csiweb.pospal.co.uk/csi-content/uploads/2021/01/Cicely-Saunders-Manifesto-A4-multipage_Jan2021-2.pdf

[2] Saunders C. Watch with me. Nursing Times. 1965;**61**(48):1615-1617

[3] Saunders C, Baines M, Dunlop R. Living with Dying: A Guide to Palliative Care. Oxford: Oxford University Press; 1995

[4] Saunders DC. Cicely Saunders: Selected Writings 1958-2004. Oxford: Oxford University Press; 2006

[5] Miller P. Dedication: Honoring Balfour Michal Morgan Mount—The Father of North American Palliative Care [Internet]. 2019. Available from: https://www.surgical.theclinics.com/action/showPdf?pii=S0039-6109%2819%2930058-1

[6] WHO Definition of Palliative Care [Internet]. 2023. Available from: https://www.who.int/europe/news-room/fact-sheets/item/palliative-care

[7] Sudnow D. Passing on. New Jersey: Prentice-Hall; 1967

[8] Knaul F, Radbruch L, Connor S, de Lima L, Arreola-Ornelas H, Mendez Carniado O. How many adults and children are in need of palliative care worldwide. In: Global Atlas of Palliative Care. 2nd ed. London: Worldwide Hospice and Palliative Care Alliance (WHPCA) and the World Health Organization (WHO); 2020. Available from: https://www.palliativecare.in/wp-content/uploads/2020/10/Global-Atlas-2nd-Edition-2020.pdf

[9] Clark D. Between hope and acceptance: The medicalisation of dying. BMJ. 2002;**324**(7342):905-907

[10] Porter R. The Greatest Benefit to Mankind: A Medical History of Humanity (The Norton History of Science). London: WW Norton & Company; 1999

[11] James N, Field D. The routinization of hospice: Charisma and bureaucratization. Social Science and Medicine. 1992;**34**(12):1363-1375

[12] Du Bobaly S. Cicely Saunders-the Founder of the Modern Hospice Movement. London: Hodder and Saughton; 2007

[13] Clark D. Total pain', disciplinary power and the body in the work of Cicely Saunders, 1958-1967. Social Science and Medicine. 1999;**49**(6):727-736

[14] Haraldsdottir E. The constraints of the ordinary: 'being with 'in the context of end-of-life nursing care. International Journal of Palliative Nursing. 2011;**17**(5):245-250

[15] Kearney M. A Place of Healing: Working with Suffering in Living and Dying. Oxford: Oxford University Press; 2000

[16] Clark D, Seymour J. Reflections on Palliative Care. Maidenhead: The Open University Press; 1999

[17] Schroeder K, Lorenz K. Nursing and the future of palliative care. Asia-Pacific Journal of Oncology Nursing. 2018;**5**(1):4-8

[18] Larkin P. Shaping new thinking in palliative nursing. International Journal of Palliative Nursing. 2007;**13**(8):364

[19] Robinson J, Gott M, Gardiner C, Ingleton C. Specialist palliative care nursing and the philosophy of palliative care: A critical discussion. International Journal of Palliative Nursing. 2017;**23**(7):352-358

[20] Moran S, Bailey ME, Doody O. Role and contribution of the nurse in caring for patients with palliative care needs: A scoping review. PLoS ONE. 2024;**19**(8):e0307188

[21] Dobrina R, Tenze M, Palese A. An overview of hospice and palliative care nursing models and theories. International Journal of Palliative Nursing. 2014;**20**(2):75-81

[22] Chochinov HM, Hack T, Hassard T, Kristjanson LJ, McClement S, Harlos M. Dignity therapy: A novel psychotherapeutic intervention for patients near the end of life. Journal of Clinical Oncology. 2005;**23**(24):5520-5525

[23] Abel J, Kellehear A, Karapliagou A. Palliative care-the new essentials. Annals of Palliative Medicine. 2018;**7**(supp2):s3-s14

[24] Gyllensten H, Björkman I, Jakobsson Ung E, Ekman I, Jakobsson S. A national research centre for the evaluation and implementation of person-centred care: Content from the first interventional studies. Health Expectations. 2020;**23**(5):1362-1375

[25] Phelan A, McCormack B, Dewing J, Brown D, Cardiff S, Cook NF, et al. Review of Developments in Person-Centred Healthcare. Notodeen, Norway: USN Open Archive; 2020. Available from: https://openarchive.usn.no/usn-xmlui/handle/11250/2753283

[26] van der Eerden M, Csikos A, Busa C, Hughes S, Radbruch L, Menten J, et al. Experiences of patients, family and professional caregivers with Integrated Palliative Care in Europe: Protocol for an international, multicenter, prospective, mixed method study. BMC Palliative Care. 2014;**13**:1-9

[27] McCormack B, McCance. The person-centred practice framework. In: McCormack B, McCance T, Bulley C, Brown D, McMillan A, Martin S, editors. Fundamentals of Person-Centred Healthcare Practice. Chichester: John Wiley & Sons; 2021. pp. 23-32

[28] Lannie A, Haraldsdottir E, Spiller J. Palliative and end of life care services. In: McCormack B, McCance T, Bulley C, Brown D, McMillan A, Martin S, editors. Fundamentals of Person-Centred Healthcare Practice. Chichester: John Wiley & Sons; 2021. pp. 257-264

[29] Leibing A. Entangled matters—Alzheimer's, interiority, and the 'unflattening' of the world. Culture, Medicine, and Psychiatry. 2008;**32**:177-193

[30] Seedhouse D. Ethics: The Heart of Health Care. New Jersey: John Wiley & Sons; 2008

[31] McCormack B, McCance T, editors. Person-Centred Practice in Nursing and Health Care: Theory and Practice. New Jersey: John Wiley & Sons; 2016

[32] Murray SA, Kendall M, Boyd K, Sheikh A. Illness trajectories and palliative care. BMJ. 2005;**330**(7498):1007-1011

[33] Haraldsdottir E, Lloyd A, Bijak M, Milton L, Finucane AM. Inpatient hospice admissions. Who is admitted and why: A mixed-method prospective study. Palliative Care and Social Practice. 2023;**17**:26323524231182724

[34] Richardson H, Cooper M. Nursing Can be Change Agents in End-of-Life Care. 2021. Available from: https://cdn.ps.emap.com/wp-content/uploads/sites/3/2021/03/010-011_NT_MAR21.pdf

[35] Franks PJ, Salisbury C, Bosanquet N, Wilkinson EK, Kite S, Naysmith A, et al. The level of need for palliative care: A systematic review of the literature. Palliative Medicine. 2000;**14**(2):93-104

[36] NHS. NIHR. An Independent Review of NIHR Research on End of Life Care Services. 2015. Available from: https://evidence.nihr.ac.uk/wp-content/uploads/2020/03/Better-endings-FINAL-WEB.pdf

Chapter 5

Perspective Chapter: Palliative Care in Nigeria – Perspectives, Challenges, and Barriers

Kafayat Oyinlade Mahmoud and Oyinlola Oluwagbemiga

Abstract

As global awareness of palliative care expands, regions like Nigeria continue to face challenges in initiating conversations on palliative care, end-of-life planning, and advanced directives. This hesitation limits a deeper understanding of how socio-cultural factors shape the perceptions and experiences of older adults and their families in Nigeria regarding palliative care. This chapter explores the disparate meanings and preparations surrounding palliative care and end-of-life practices across Nigeria's major ethnic groups *(Yoruba, Igbo, and Hausa)*. It examines the impact of human rights concerns in the context of palliative care, especially given the absence of comprehensive policy frameworks across many African regions. Additionally, this chapter addresses the structural and practical challenges in implementing palliative care and highlights opportunities to develop an Afrocentric approach. This approach is rooted in the lived realities of older adults and their families, aiming to provide culturally resonant and ethically sound care within Nigeria's unique socio-cultural landscape.

Keywords: palliative care, end-of-life planning, older adults, afrocentric-approach, Nigerian healthcare

1. Introduction

Palliative and end-of-life care hold profound cultural significance across geopolitical regions of Nigeria, and are connected to the interplay between traditional beliefs, familial responsibilities, and the healthcare system's capacity to support individuals facing terminal illnesses [1–3]. While the concept of palliative care has gained international recognition as an essential component of comprehensive healthcare, its interpretation and implementation within the Nigerian context diverges notably from global understandings [4, 5]. Much of this divergence is rooted in religious and cultural perceptions of illness and death, the structure of the Nigerian healthcare system, and the essential roles of families and communities in caregiving. This book chapter offers insights into the unique perspectives that shape the effective implementation of palliative care in Nigeria and potential solutions informed by the Afrocentric realities of Nigerian families.

The Nigerian healthcare system primarily focuses on curative care, with limited attention to end-of-life care. Indeed, the limited availability of palliative care services, exacerbated by inadequate funding, lack of trained professionals, and insufficient infrastructure, reflects a broader issue of under-resourced healthcare systems in many African countries [6, 7]. While global frameworks, such as the World Health Organization's call for universal health coverage, include palliative care, Nigeria has yet to implement comprehensive national policies that integrate palliative care into the healthcare system [6, 8]. This policy vacuum results in inadequate funding, insufficient healthcare infrastructure, and a lack of essential medications, such as opioids, needed to manage pain effectively. Additionally, the formal healthcare system has been slow to integrate palliative care services, partly due to inadequate awareness among healthcare professionals and the general population [1, 5, 9]. These factors, consequently, contribute to delayed referrals and misconceptions about palliative care, often equating it with a "death sentence" rather than a supportive, holistic approach to patient care. These challenges are exacerbated by the complexity of Nigeria's healthcare system, which struggles to meet the demands of an aging population amid socioeconomic disparities, cultural expectations of care, and inadequate public health funding [2].

From a cultural perspective, palliative care in Nigeria is also influenced by deep-rooted beliefs about death, illness, and family roles in caregiving. Traditional African concepts of illness, such as spiritual or ancestral causes, often shape care preferences, and palliative care is sometimes viewed as contradictory to cultural values that emphasize curative efforts [8, 10]. This cultural reticence hinders the implementation of advanced care planning and can lead to conflict between healthcare providers and families who may prefer traditional healing methods or have unrealistic expectations of curative treatments. Furthermore, the communal nature of caregiving, grounded in the Ubuntu philosophy, suggests that family and community involvement is critical in end-of-life care, yet this can also place heavy burdens on families, particularly in the absence of formalized support systems [11–13]. Exploring those unique cultural beliefs and practices that either support and/or obstruct the implementation of palliative care in Nigeria is warranted.

Uniquely, this chapter critiques the policy landscape surrounding palliative care in Nigeria, which lacks comprehensive national guidelines or strategic frameworks. Despite global efforts to promote palliative care as a human right, Nigeria's policy environment reflects a broader underinvestment in chronic disease management and end-of-life care [5, 14]. The absence of integrated palliative care policies is compounded by inconsistent government commitment and limited collaboration among healthcare sectors, non-governmental organizations, and international bodies. This chapter argues that policy reforms that advocate a paradigm shift, recognizing palliative care not only as a clinical necessity, but as an essential component of health equity and human dignity in Nigeria.

2. Cultural perspective of illness, dying, and death in Nigeria

Nigeria is home to over two-hundred and fifty (250) ethnic groups with unique traditions, beliefs, and practices surrounding illness, dying, and death [15, 16]. While the cultural meanings and perspective of illness conditions are still empirically emerging, the nuance difference between major cultures (Yoruba, Igbo and Hausa), alongside the major religious organization Christianity, Islam, and indigenous religions, significantly shapes the construction of palliative care and terminal illness in Nigeria [17–19]. For instance, among the Yoruba people, predominantly found in southwestern Nigeria, illness and death are viewed through a spiritual lens [10, 20]. In the cosmology of Yoruba, life is cyclical, with death perceived as a transition to another phase of existence, just like "Àkódà" (*origin*) and "Àsè" (*spiritual authority*) signifies the belief that a good death, achieved through appropriate rites and rituals, ensures a seamless passage to the ancestral realm [21, 22]. While this belief shapes the Yoruba approach to palliative care, these culturally rich perspectives are often a misfit with Western biomedical approaches, which focuses on curative medicine and individual autonomy, sidelining communal decision-making processes and the spiritual dimensions of care have dominated healthcare systems in Nigeria. Many Yoruba families often seek the counsel of elders or traditional healers for end-of-life decisions, and healthcare professionals in formal settings may dismiss palliative practices as unscientific [23, 24]. In southeastern Nigeria, the Igbo people of Nigeria, death (*onwu*) is not merely the cessation of life but a transition to the ancestral realm (*ndi ichie*) [25, 26]. The care for the dying emphasizes dignity, respect, and the spiritual preparation of the individual, which allows families to take an active role in providing emotional and physical support, a process often guided by traditional healers (*dibia*) and religious rituals [27, 28]. Although the Igbo and Yoruba cultures shares some similarities, such as the belief in continuity between worlds and the communal nature of caregiving, the Yoruba concept of *ikú* (death) is more closely tied to destiny (*ayanmo*), with greater emphasis on the deceased's *orí* (spiritual essence).

For the Hausa, who predominantly reside in northern Nigeria, the notion of *kyautata rayuwa* (improving life) emphasizes the importance of holistic care that addresses the physical, emotional, and spiritual well-being of the individual. Care for the terminally ill often takes place within the *zaman iyali* (family structure), where relatives, particularly women, play crucial caregiving roles [29, 30]. Islam, which is central to Hausa identity, profoundly influences perceptions of death and dying in situations where the beliefs about *ƙaddara* (destiny) and *iman* (faith) shape attitudes toward illness, reinforces acceptance of life's impermanence [31, 32]. The recitation of *du'a* (prayers) and reliance on *al'ummar musulmai* (the Muslim community) for spiritual support are integral to end-of-life practices [31, 32]. While death is approached with resignation to divine will, misconceptions about *kulawar rashin lafiya na ƙarshe* (end-of-life care) persist, with some associating it with abandonment or hopelessness. Although there are cultural differences in perspectives about palliative care, the Hausa approach tends to remain more explicitly tied to Islamic lens, which may downplay ritualistic expressions compared to the celebratory and symbolic aspects observed in Yoruba traditions [17, 33]. Additionally, while Igbo practices may sometimes integrate divination to address spiritual concerns about illness and death, Hausa traditions emphasize unwavering reliance on Allah's will, reflecting a theological divergence.

Despite these differences, the rich cultural diversity of Nigeria reveals the complexity of integrating palliative care practices that align with local beliefs and traditions. Although the Yoruba, Igbo, and Hausa cultures differ in their spiritual frameworks and caregiving approaches, all three similarly emphasize communal involvement and the spiritual dimensions of care—elements often overlooked by Western biomedical models. These cultural paradigms also challenge Eurocentric emphasis on individual autonomy, urging a more inclusive approach to palliative care. Indeed, an Afrocentric approach such as Ubuntu that embraces values that fosters a synergy between traditional and biomedical practices that honor the dignity, spirituality, and communal essence of end-of-life care is eminently warranted.

3. Human rights of older adults in death preparation in Nigeria

Although Nigeria and several African countries are signatories to the United Nations Charter on human rights and the African Charter on the rights of older adults, emphasis on palliative care and end of life care is either missing or still at infancy stages in most of African countries. The Nigerian constitution recognizes the right of all citizens to health care in Section (16)2;17 of the 1999 constitution of the Federal Republic of Nigeria, yet specific legislation regarding palliative and end of life care remains missing. Furthermore, while the Nigeria government has a protocol for improving well-being of older adults in the region such as found in the National Aging policy, a well-mapped out process of supporting older adults to make informed decision about their lives, including palliative and end of life care, remains unavailable [34].

In 2020, the Nigerian government, through the Federal Ministry of Humanitarian Affairs, Disaster Management, and Social Development, designed the National Policy on Aging to address the well-being of older persons [35, 36]. Premised on the 1999 Constitution of the Federal Republic of Nigeria, this policy envisions a society where older persons are guaranteed security, independence, participation, comprehensive care, self-fulfillment, and dignity [37]. These objectives align with global human rights frameworks, which emphasize the right to health and well-being at all stages of life. However, despite this progressive policy, the reality remains stark—long-term care systems, including palliative and end-of-life care, are underdeveloped and inaccessible to most Nigerians. To date, only 10 facilities provide palliative care nationwide, with five associated with tertiary hospitals. These facilities are disproportionately located in the southwestern region, with one each in the southern (Port Harcourt) and southeastern (Enugu) regions, leaving vast areas in the northern and western regions underserved [35]. The inadequacy of palliative care services reflects broader structural inequalities, including the role of privileged, socioeconomic status, and education in determining access to information and affordability of these services. For many families, who are often the primary caregivers for chronically ill older adults, the lack of awareness about palliative care further exacerbates the burden of care [1, 15].

While absence of specific laws and enforceable policies on palliative and end-of-life care represents a violation of the basic human rights of older adults, lack of structured systems denies them access to equitable, affordable, and quality care, undermining their right to live and die with dignity. In addition, when older adults are deprived of adequate information or support to make decisions about their own care, particularly at the palliative and end-of-life stages, a fundamental breach of their human rights occurs. Central to these rights is the principle of autonomy, which upholds each individual's freedom to make informed choices about their own body, treatment options, and overall well-being [38]. Withholding crucial information—such as the risks, benefits, and alternatives of proposed interventions—healthcare providers, institutions, or family members serve to undermine the autonomy, reducing older adults to passive recipients of care rather than respected agents of their own destinies.

This violation transcends medical ethics and becomes a broader issue of human dignity. For instance, when older adults cannot participate meaningfully in decisions about pain management, life support, or comfort measures, they are deprived of their right to self-determination. Such paternalistic approaches may result in fear, anxiety, and a deep sense of powerlessness [39, 40]. It also perpetuates inequities, as lack of access to clear, culturally sensitive information disproportionately affects those with fewer resources or lower literacy levels. In extreme cases, families or institutions may override older adults' expressed wishes, a systemic discrimination that views them as less capable or deserving of respect. Ensuring adequate information, counseling, and psychological support for older persons safeguards their right to decide how and where they spend their remaining days.

This chapter advocates the proposal of legislative reforms, resource allocation, and public education which uphold the principles of justice, equity, and compassion in the care of older adults that require palliative and end of life care. Although Afrocentric practices such as Ubuntu are still at the infancy stage in most African regions, its emphasis on community, interdependence, and respect for elders could offer positively support older adults in making informed decisions at the palliative and end-of-life stages [33, 41]. These principles align with the ethical rule of doing good, or beneficence, which prioritizes the well-being and dignity of individuals. However, without adequate information or support, these values can inadvertently lead to decision substitution, where family or community members impose their preferences, believing they are acting in the older person's best interests [42, 43]. This risks violating autonomy and perpetuating harm, as it denies the older adult their rightful voice. Balancing Afrocentric values with a rights-based approach ensures that cultural practices enhance, rather than compromise, informed decision-making and individual agency.

4. Barriers to providing palliative care in Nigeria

As discussed in previous sections, palliative care in Nigeria is shaped by cultural, religious, and social beliefs about illness, death, and dying, which may present distinct challenges. Illness is often perceived through a spiritual, traditional, and communal lens [20], and palliative care could be seen as "giving up" on curative treatment, which conflicts with cultural values of hope and faith in healing [44, 45]. As a result, families may resist palliative care, perceiving it as abandoning the patient. Additionally, cultural stigma against discussing death further complicate early engagement with end-of-life care, as many Nigerians believe that speaking about death invites it, deterring families from planning or seeking palliative support [3, 17].

Access to palliative care highlights significant rural–urban disparities. Urban areas, though limited, offer hospitals with palliative care units or specialists [4, 46]. In contrast, rural regions often lack basic healthcare infrastructure, leaving families reliant on underfunded primary healthcare centers or home-based care. These families must frequently travel long distances to access necessary services, exacerbating inequities in pain relief and quality end-of-life care [17, 23]. Furthermore, healthcare professionals are often unprepared to address these challenges. Nigeria's medical curricula rarely covers palliative care, particularly with regard to cultural sensitivity, leaving providers ill-equipped to handle sensitive discussions about advanced directives, treatment discontinuation, or hospice care [5, 47]. This gap fosters mistrust and dissatisfaction among families, who may feel their values are disregarded.

Finally, home-based care imposes significant financial burdens on families. Costs for medications, supplies, and transportation are often prohibitive, compounded by limited access to essential pain management drugs like morphine due to regulatory barriers [1, 4]. Ethical dilemmas further hinder palliative care delivery. Pain management is constrained by fears of opioid addiction and regulatory restrictions, leading to unnecessary patient suffering [1, 48]. Decisions about life support and advanced directives are similarly fraught, as families may view withdrawing life support as morally unacceptable. Healthcare providers must navigate these conflicts between professional guidelines and cultural expectations, often at the expense of patient autonomy.

5. Opportunities for integrating a cultural appropriate model of palliative care in Nigeria

A culturally sensitive approach to palliative care in Nigeria offers a meaningful way to improve end-of-life care by respecting and incorporating the country's rich cultural, religious, and social diversity. This model acknowledges the important roles of traditional healers, religious leaders, and community structures while addressing gaps in awareness and providing targeted training for healthcare professionals.

5.1 Traditional healers

Traditional healers are central to healthcare in rural Nigeria, where access to modern medical services is limited. As trusted members of their communities, they are often the first point of contact for people seeking care [1, 49, 50]. Training traditional healers in basic palliative care skills—such as pain management and emotional support—can empower them to provide care that aligns with cultural expectations while building bridges to modern palliative care services.

5.2 Religious leaders

Religious leaders hold profound influence over beliefs about illness, death, and dying in Nigeria. Their voices can address widespread misconceptions, such as the idea that palliative care signifies a lack of faith or hope [31]. By equipping religious leaders with the tools to offer spiritual guidance consistent with palliative care, families can be encouraged to seek timely care and engage in open, meaningful conversations about end-of-life decisions.

5.3 Community structures

Local councils, women's groups, and other community organizations play a powerful role in shaping public attitudes and behavior. These groups, deeply embedded in communities, can drive awareness campaigns, organize training, and create support networks for those facing serious illness [17]. Their involvement ensures that care is tailored to local realities and rooted in trust.

5.4 Education and awareness

A major challenge in Nigeria is the lack of understanding about what palliative care is and how it can benefit individuals and families. Public education campaigns, conducted in local languages and framed within cultural norms, can break down barriers and correct misconceptions [4]. Strategies such as radio programs, community workshops, and storytelling sessions can explain palliative care as a compassionate, holistic approach to physical, emotional, and spiritual well-being.

5.5 Healthcare provider training

Healthcare professionals need culturally informed training to meet the complex needs of patients and families at the end of life. Medical curricula should incorporate lessons on cultural competence, particularly in handling sensitive topics such as pain relief and advanced directives. Collaborations between hospitals and community stakeholders can further enhance trust and improve quality-of-care delivery.

6. Conclusion

In this chapter, we critically examine the unique challenges associated with adopting and implementing Eurocentric palliative care within Nigeria's diverse sociocultural landscape. Yoruba, Igbo, and Hausa traditions, with their emphasis on communal bonds and spiritual care, contrast sharply with global frameworks that prioritize individual autonomy. Bridging these differing perspectives requires the integration of Afrocentric values, such as Ubuntu, alongside legislative reforms. Traditional healers, religious leaders, and community groups play a crucial role as culturally informed allies, contributing valuable insights to enrich care delivery and strengthen family engagement. Equally essential are policies that uphold the human rights of older adults, ensuring access to informed decision-making, effective pain management, and dignity in care. Collaboration among stakeholders—including policymakers, healthcare professionals, religious institutions, and civil society—is critical to developing targeted programs, expanding specialized training, and removing regulatory barriers to essential medications. Sustained investment in research, policy dialog, and resources is indispensable for fostering an evolving palliative care paradigm that prioritizes compassion, equity, and cultural relevance in Nigeria's healthcare system.

Author details

Kafayat Oyinlade Mahmoud[1*] and Oyinlola Oluwagbemiga[2]

1 Centre for Social Innovations, Boston University, Boston, USA

2 School of Social Work, McGill University, Montreal, Canada

*Address all correspondence to: kmahmoud@bu.edu

References

[1] Afolabi OA, Nkhoma K, Soyannwo O, Aje A, Ogunniyi A, Harding R, et al. Integrated primary palliative Care in Nigeria-Perspectives of patients, families and providers. Journal of Pain and Symptom Management. 2022;**64**(4):319-329. DOI: 10.1016/j.jpainsymman.2022.06.019

[2] Gysels M, Pell C, Straus L, Pool R. End of life care in sub-Saharan Africa: A systematic review of the qualitative literature. BMC Palliative Care. 2011;**10**(1):6. DOI: 10.1186/1472-684X-10-6

[3] Omoyeni E, Gwyther L. Assessing the palliative care needs of elderly patients seen at The University College Hospital, Ibadan, Nigeria (TH321A). Journal of Pain and Symptom Management. 2018;**55**(2):571-572. DOI: 10.1016/j.jpainsymman.2017.12.027

[4] Agom DA, Onyeka TC, Iheanacho PN, Ominyi J. Barriers to the provision and utilization of palliative Care in Africa: A rapid scoping review. Indian Journal of Palliative Care. 2021;**27**(1):3-17. DOI: 10.4103/IJPC.IJPC_355_20

[5] Ogbenna A, Drane D, Crowe AN, Oyedele O, Hauser J, Soyannwo O, et al. Building the Nigerian palliative care workforce: An interdisciplinary distance learning training program. Annals of Global Health. 2022;**88**(1). DOI: 10.5334/aogh.3744

[6] Ntizimira CR, Nkurikiyimfura JL, Mukeshimana O, Ngizwenayo S, Mukasahaha D, Clancy C. Palliative Care in Africa: A Global Challenge; 2014. DOI: 10.3332/ecancer.2014.493

[7] Palumbo N, Tilly A, Namisango E, Ntizimira C, Thambo L, Chikasema M, et al. Palliative care in Malawi: A scoping review. BMC Palliative Care. 2023;**22**(1):146. DOI: 10.1186/s12904-023-01264-8

[8] Luyirika E, Lohman D, Ali Z, Atieno M, Mahenge A, Mmbando P, et al. Progress update: Palliative care development between 2017 and 2020 in five African countries. Journal of Pain and Symptom Management. 2022;**63**(5):729-736. DOI: 10.1016/j.jpainsymman.2021.12.026

[9] Adenipekun A, Onibokun A, Elumelu TN, Soyannwo OA. Knowledge and attitudes of terminally ill patients and their family to palliative care and hospice services in Nigeria. Nigerian Journal of Clinical Practice. 2005;**8**(1):19-22

[10] Jegede A, Adegoke O. Advance directive in end of life decision-making among Yoruba of south-western, Nigeria. BEOnline Journal of the Center for Bioethics and Research. 2016;**3**(4):41-67. DOI: 10.20541/beonline.2016.0008

[11] Court L, Olivier J. Approaches to integrating palliative care into African health systems: A qualitative systematic review. Health Policy and Planning. 2020;**35**(8):1053-1069. DOI: 10.1093/heapol/czaa026

[12] Kimani KN, Namukwaya E, Grant L, Murray SA. Cancer and palliative care in Africa. European Journal of Cancer Care. 2017;**26**(1):e12655. DOI: 10.1111/ecc.12655

[13] Rhee JY, Garralda E, Namisango E, Luyirika E, de Lima L, Powell RA, et al. The african palliative care association (APCA) Atlas of palliative care development in Africa: A comparative analysis. The Lancet Global Health.

2018;**6**:S21. DOI: 10.1016/S2214-109X(18)30150-5

[14] Doobay-Persaud A, Solchanyk D, Fleming O, Patel N, Drane D, Hauser J, et al. Palliative care challenges in Nigeria: A qualitative study of interprofessional perceptions. Journal of Pain and Symptom Management. 2023;**65**(1):e1-e5. DOI: 10.1016/j.jpainsymman.2022.10.002

[15] Adejoh SO, Boele F, Akeju D, Dandadzi A, Nabirye E, Namisango E, et al. The role, impact, and support of informal caregivers in the delivery of palliative care for patients with advanced cancer: A multi-country qualitative study. Palliative Medicine. 2021;**35**(3):552-562. DOI: 10.1177/0269216320974925

[16] Eyetsemitan F. Cultural interpretation of dying and death in a non-western society: The case of Nigeria. Online Readings in Psychology and Culture. 2002;**3**(2):4-10. DOI: 10.9707/2307-0919.1090

[17] Cadmus EO, Oyinlola O, Obadare A, Adebusoye LA, Mahmoud K. Knowledge and perception of older adults toward end of life and advanced directive in Nigeria. Palliative and Supportive Care. 2024:1-8. DOI: 10.1017/S1478951524001615

[18] Ekore RI, Lanre-Abass B. African cultural concept of death and the idea of advance care directives. Indian Journal of Palliative Care. 2016;**22**(4):369-372. DOI: 10.4103/0973-1075.191741

[19] Lanre-Abass BA. Cultural differences in advance directives relating to end of life decision making. Prajñā Vihāra: Journal of Philosophy and Religion. 2008;**9**(1):Article 1. Available from: http://www.assumptionjournal.au.edu/index.php/PrajnaVihara/article/view/1261

[20] Jegede AS. The Yoruba cultural construction of health and illness. Nordic Journal of African Studies. 2002;**11**(3):Article 3. DOI: 10.53228/njas.v11i3.345

[21] Olomola I. Contradictions in Yoruba folk beliefs concerning post-life existence: The ado example; 1988. DOI: 10.3406/jafr.1988.2255

[22] Ọsanyìnbí ỌB, Falana K. An evaluation of the Akure Yorùbá traditional belief in reincarnation. Open Journal of Philosophy. 2016;**6**(01):59-67. DOI: 10.4236/ojpp.2016.61007

[23] Cadmus EO, Adebusoye LA, Olowookere OO, Olusegun AT, Oyinlola O, Adeleke RO, et al. Older persons' perceptions about advanced directives and end of life issues in a geriatric care setting in southwestern Nigeria. The Pan African Medical Journal. 2019;**32**:64. DOI: 10.11604/pamj.2019.32.64.17117

[24] Esther Oyebade O, Oyinlola O, Asenjo Palma C. Difficult but achievable: Medical social workers' experiences transiting older adults from hospital care to nursing home in Nigeria. Social Work in Health Care. 2024;**0**(0):1-15. DOI: 10.1080/00981389.2024.2324859

[25] Stefanovics EA, He H, Cavalcanti M, Neto H, Ofori-Atta A, Leddy M, et al. Witchcraft and biopsychosocial causes of mental illness: Attitudes and beliefs about mental illness among health professionals in five countries. The Journal of Nervous and Mental Disease. 2016;**204**(3):169-174. DOI: 10.1097/NMD.0000000000000422

[26] Nwoye CM. Igbo cultural and religious worldview: An insider's perspective. International Journal of Sociology and Anthropology. 2011;**3**(9):304-317

[27] Daaleman TP, Usher BM, Williams SW, Rawlings J, Hanson LC. An exploratory study of spiritual Care at the end of life. Annals of Family Medicine. 2008;**6**(5):406. DOI: 10.1370/afm.883

[28] Hinshaw DB. The spiritual needs of the dying patient. Journal of the American College of Surgeons. 2002;**195**(4):565. DOI: 10.1016/S1072-7515(02)01328-5

[29] Abdullahi R. Self-Concept and Cultural Change in the Hausa of Nigeria. Ibadan: Ibadan University Press; 1977

[30] Abubakar MS, Musa AM, Ahmed A, Hussaini IM. The perception and practice of traditional medicine in the treatment of cancers and inflammations by the Hausa and Fulani tribes of northern Nigeria. Journal of Ethnopharmacology. 2007;**111**(3):625-629. DOI: 10.1016/j.jep.2007.01.011

[31] Badru AI, Kanmodi KK. Palliative care awareness amongst religious leaders and seminarians: A Nigerian study. The Pan African Medical Journal. 2017;**28**(259):Article 259. DOI: 10.11604/pamj.2017.28.259.14010

[32] Henry D, Kemp C. Culture and the end of life: Nigerians. Journal of Hospice and Palliative Nursing. 2002;**4**(2):111

[33] Oyinlola O, Gyan C, Mugumbate JR. Ubuntu: A Cultural Method of Dementia Caregiving in Africa. The Ubuntu Practitioner: Social Work Perspectives. Switzerland; 2023. p. 384

[34] United Nations. Department of Economic and Social Affairs, Population Division. World Population Ageing 2019: Highlights (ST/ESA/SER.A/430); 2019

[35] Mbam KC, Halvorsen CJ, Okoye UO. Aging in Nigeria: A growing population of older adults requires the implementation of national aging policies. The Gerontologist. 2022;**62**(9):1243-1250. DOI: 10.1093/geront/gnac121

[36] Ogunyemi AO, Balogun MR, Ojo AE, Welch SB, Onasanya OO, Yesufu VO, et al. Provider and facility readiness for age-friendly health services for older adults in primary health care centres in southwest, Nigeria. PLOS Global Public Health. 2023;**3**(8):e0001411. DOI: 10.1371/journal.pgph.0001411

[37] Lamai S. FG Approves National Policy On Ageing For Older Persons In Nigeria. Federal Ministry of Information and National Orientation; 2021. Available from: https://fmino.gov.ng/fg-approves-national-policy-on-ageing-for-older-persons-in-nigeria/

[38] Entwistle VA, Carter SM, Cribb A, McCaffery K. Supporting patient autonomy: The importance of clinician-patient relationships. Journal of General Internal Medicine. 2010;**25**(7):741-745. DOI: 10.1007/s11606-010-1292-2

[39] Garrett SB, Nicosia F, Thompson N, Miaskowski C, Ritchie CS. Barriers and facilitators to older adults' use of nonpharmacologic approaches for chronic pain: A person-focused model. Pain. 2021;**162**(11):2769-2779. DOI: 10.1097/j.pain.0000000000002260

[40] Ross MM, Carswell A, Hing M, Hollingworth G, Dalziel WB. Seniors' decision making about pain management. Journal of Advanced Nursing. 2001;**35**(3):442-451. DOI: 10.1046/j.1365-2648.2001.01859.x

[41] Balestrery JE. Ubuntu and Social Work: Advancing a Global Lens and Language in Healthcare. The Ubuntu Practitioner: Social Work Perspectives. Switzerland; 2023. p. 626

[42] Hegde S, Ellajosyula R. Capacity issues and decision-making in dementia. Annals of Indian Academy of Neurology. 2016;**19**(Suppl 1):S34. DOI: 10.4103/0972-2327.192890

[43] Schroeder D, Chatfield K, Singh M, Chennells R, Herissone-Kelly P. The four values framework: Fairness, respect, care and honesty. In: Schroeder D, Chatfield K, Singh M, Chennells R, Herissone-Kelly P, editors. Equitable Research Partnerships: A Global Code of Conduct to Counter Ethics Dumping. Cham: Springer International Publishing; 2019. pp. 13-26. DOI: 10.1007/978-3-030-15745-6_3

[44] Adebayo PB, Abayomi O, Johnson PO, Oloyede T, Oyelekan AAA. Breaking bad news in clinical setting—Health professionals' experience and perceived competence in Southwestern Nigeria: A cross sectional study. Annals of African Medicine. 2013;**12**(4):205-211. DOI: 10.4103/1596-3519.122687

[45] Nissim R, Flora DB, Cribbie RA, Zimmermann C, Gagliese L, Rodin G. Factor structure of the Beck Hopelessness Scale in individuals with advanced cancer. Psycho-Oncology. 2010;**19**(3): 255-263. DOI: 10.1002/pon.1540

[46] Idemili-Aronu N, Onyeka TC, Okenwa UJ, Jemisenia JO, Okoli IA, Olawepo JO, et al. Knowledge, attitudes, and barriers: Palliative Care services for women with HIV in resource-limited settings. BMC Palliative Care. 2024;**23**(1):227. DOI: 10.1186/s12904-024-01558-5

[47] Oji N, Onyeka T, Soyannwo O, Paal P, Elsner F. Perspectives, perceived self-efficacy, and preparedness of newly qualified physicians' in practising palliative care—A qualitative study. BMC Palliative Care. 2022;**21**(1):141. DOI: 10.1186/s12904-022-01028-w

[48] Magboh VO, Saba OA, Krause R, Forget P. Barriers to Optimal Management of Cancer Pain in Sub-Saharan. Africa: A Scoping Review; 2023. DOI: 10.3332/ecancer.2023.1650

[49] Anjorin O, Hassan Wada Y. Impact of traditional healers in the provision of mental health services in Nigeria. Annals of Medicine and Surgery. 2022;**82**:104755. DOI: 10.1016/j.amsu.2022.104755

[50] Asuzu CC, Akin-Odanye EO, Asuzu MC, Holland J. A socio-cultural study of traditional healers role in African health care. Infectious Agents and Cancer. 2019;**14**(1):15. DOI: 10.1186/s13027-019-0232-y

Section 2

Assessment and Evaluation

Chapter 6

Toward a Global Assessment of Quality of Life in Pediatric Palliative Care: A Multidisciplinary Approach

Laia Riera-Negre, Maria Rosa Rosselló and Sebastià Verger

Abstract

The PACOPED QL is an innovative, multidimensional tool designed to evaluate the quality of life of children in palliative care and those with complex chronic illnesses. It addresses a critical need for comprehensive assessments that go beyond clinical aspects to include emotional, social, and educational dimensions. Developed through a collaborative and multidisciplinary process, the PACOPED QL captures eight key areas of QoL, including physical and emotional well-being, social inclusion, and personal development. The instrument's applicability spans health care, educational, and community settings, offering a practical framework to inform personalized care, promote inclusion, and guide interventions. Its multidimensional design enables professionals from diverse disciplines to address various facets of the child's life, fostering coordinated efforts that enhance overall well-being. Additionally, the PACOPED QL has the potential to influence public policies by providing evidence-based insights into the needs of this vulnerable population. Its ultimate goal is to empower caregivers and professionals to support children holistically, ensuring they experience not only survival but also meaningful, fulfilling lives.

Keywords: pediatric palliative care, quality of life, multidimensional assessment, chronic illnesses, holistic care

1. Introduction

Quality of life (QoL) has emerged as a fundamental construct in research on human well-being, becoming particularly relevant in vulnerable populations such as children and adolescents with chronic and life-threatening illnesses [1–4]. The World Health Organization [5] defines QoL as an individual's perception of their position in life, within the context of the culture and value systems in which they live, and in relation to their goals, expectations, standards, and concerns. This definition highlights the subjective and multidimensional nature of QoL, which extends beyond the mere absence of disease or discomfort. In the context of Pediatric Palliative Care (PPC), assessing QoL takes on a critical dimension, as patients face not only physical challenges but also psychological, social, and educational issues that profoundly impact their well-being and that of their families [6–8].

In recent decades, PPC has evolved to more comprehensively address the needs of children with life-threatening or life-limiting illnesses [9, 10]. Unlike adult palliative care, the pediatric approach presents specific particularities due to the variability of diseases, the wide age range of patients, and the central role of the family in care [6]. The Association for Children's Palliative Care (ACT) classifies these illnesses into four groups, ranging from life-threatening conditions with the potential for curative treatment to irreversible conditions involving severe disabilities [11]. This underscores the importance of having tools capable of comprehensively evaluating the QoL of children in these diverse contexts. Although advances in medical care have significantly improved the survival of children with chronic conditions, research on the socio-educational and psychological aspects of these children has been limited [12]. Tools such as the Pediatric Quality of Life Inventory (PedsQL) and the Child Health Questionnaire (CHQ) have been widely used to assess QoL in pediatric populations. However, these tools fail to adequately capture the multidimensional and complex experiences of children in palliative care settings, where well-being extends beyond clinical aspects to encompass emotional, educational, and social needs. This highlights the critical need for a multidimensional instrument capable of evaluating various aspects of well-being, including physical, emotional, psychological, social, and educational domains.

The literature has also shown that the QoL of these patients is profoundly influenced by the quality of education and the degree of social inclusion they experience [13, 14]. Children and adolescents with life-limiting illnesses are often excluded from traditional educational settings due to their health conditions, leading to negative consequences for their emotional and social development [15–17]. Some studies emphasize the importance of inclusive educational environments to promote the participation of these children and ensure that, despite their health conditions, they have the opportunity to learn, grow, and feel part of their community [18–20].

To address these limitations, the Palliative and Complex Pediatric QoL (PACOPED QL) questionnaire was developed—an innovative, multidimensional instrument designed to assess the QoL of children in palliative care and with complex chronic illnesses. PACOPED QL is designed not only to evaluate physical well-being but also to capture key aspects such as emotional well-being, interpersonal relationships, self-determination, and patient rights. The theoretical foundation for the development of this instrument is based on the holistic model by Schalock and Verdugo [21], which has proven particularly useful for evaluating QoL in populations with disabilities and complex needs. This multidimensional approach enables a more accurate and comprehensive assessment of the well-being of the patient and their family. The development of the PACOPED QL was carried out through a collaborative and multidisciplinary process involving experts in PPC, developmental psychology, inclusive education, caregivers, healthcare professionals, and methodology specialists. This collaboration was essential to ensure that the instrument accurately reflected the unique experiences and needs of children in palliative care and that it was suitable for use in clinical, educational, and other contexts where these children are cared for. Furthermore, multicenter studies were conducted to validate the questionnaire's structure and ensure its reliability and validity across different cultural and socioeconomic contexts [22].

Therefore, building on everything discussed, this chapter will focus on the need for innovative tools that enable a comprehensive assessment of the QoL of children in PPC. The PACOPED QL not only fills an existing gap in the literature and clinical practice but also contributes to the development of a more holistic and child-centered approach, where physical, emotional, social, and educational well-being are considered inseparable parts of the care process [23]. The relevance of this instrument lies in its application across health care, educational, and other contexts that support these children, fostering a comprehensive understanding of the patient's well-being. The ultimate goal of this tool is to facilitate communication among professionals, improve personalized care planning, and ultimately promote a better QoL for children and their families in extraordinarily challenging circumstances.

2. Why did we do it? Justification

The QoL of children with chronic illnesses and life-limiting conditions is a critical aspect that requires comprehensive and multidimensional evaluation [24, 25]. PPC, unlike adult palliative care, presents unique challenges due to the wide diversity of conditions, the variability in treatment duration, and the central role of the family in care [13, 26]. These characteristics require a specific tool capable of accurately capturing all relevant aspects of the child's well-being, ensuring that the full context in which these patients live is considered [11, 27].

Despite significant advancements in medical care, attention to the QoL of children with palliative care needs remains insufficient, particularly regarding their emotional, social, and educational development [6, 13]. A review of the literature highlights the scarcity of instruments that comprehensively address the various aspects of these children's well-being, such as physical, emotional, psychological, social, and educational domains [24]. Furthermore, existing tools, such as the Pediatric QoL Inventory (PedsQL) and the Child Health Questionnaire (CHQ), while useful, do not meet the specific needs of the PPC population, which requires a deeper and more tailored evaluation.

In this context, the development of the PACOPED QL emerges as a response to this urgent need. This instrument aims not only to assess the clinical aspects of the child's well-being but also to encompass fundamental dimensions that are often overlooked, such as education, social inclusion, and self-determination. The inclusion of these dimensions reflects a holistic, child-centered approach that seeks to go beyond the illness to understand the patient as a whole and ensure a fulfilling QoL [21]. The importance of this approach becomes even more evident when considering the impact of educational and social exclusion on the well-being of children with life-limiting illnesses [28]. The PACOPED QL also holds significant relevance across clinical, educational, and community contexts. In health care, it enables professionals to gain a more comprehensive understanding of the patient's condition, facilitating personalized care and better treatment planning. In educational settings, this instrument has the potential to guide educators in creating inclusive environments and adapting pedagogical strategies to meet the specific needs of these students. Furthermore, the PACOPED QL has applications in the community sphere, fostering cooperation among various stakeholders involved in the child's well-being, such as social services, support organizations, and local communities. The multidimensionality of the PACOPED QL is one of the most innovative and necessary aspects in the evaluation of QoL in PPC [29]. This holistic approach enables the instrument to address everything from physical well-being to social inclusion and personal development, providing a more comprehensive picture of the child's condition and identifying areas for intervention to improve their QoL. The multicenter validation of the instrument and its collaborative development with experts from various disciplines enhance its applicability across different contexts and ensure its alignment with the realities of pediatric patients with complex illnesses [22].

The design of this instrument is justified as an essential tool for assessing the QoL of children in palliative care, addressing a critical gap in the care of this population. Its multidimensional design and inclusive, collaborative approach make it a valuable resource for healthcare professionals, educators, and caregivers alike. The ultimate goal is to ensure that every child, regardless of their health condition, can achieve the best possible QoL by addressing not only their physical needs but also their emotional, social, and educational well-being, thereby enabling truly patient-centered care.

3. How did we do it? Methods

The creation of the PACOPED QL questionnaire was not just an academic exercise—it was a thoughtful and much-needed effort to better understand and support the well-being of children in palliative care. The process was designed to be practical and grounded in real-life needs, always keeping the children and their families at the center. To make this possible, the project used a multidimensional and collaborative approach, ensuring the tool could be useful in many different settings, such as health care, schools, and community organizations. The focus was not just on designing the questionnaire but also on how it could be put into practice, integrated into daily care and education, and even used as a foundation for future studies and improvements.

3.1 Design of the questionnaire: A collaborative and patient-centered approach

When we set out to develop the PACOPED QL, our first step was to identify the essential dimensions that define the QoL for children with life-limiting conditions. Drawing from the theoretical framework of Schalock and Verdugo [21], we identified eight key dimensions: physical well-being, emotional well-being, interpersonal relationships, social inclusion, self-determination, rights, material well-being, and personal development. These dimensions go beyond the child's medical condition, capturing fundamental aspects of their growth as social beings and their interactions with their environment.

To ensure the questionnaire effectively addressed these dimensions, we collaborated with a multidisciplinary team. This team included experts in PPC, developmental psychology, inclusive education, and research methodology. By bringing together diverse perspectives, we made sure the questionnaire was relevant and easy to understand for everyone involved—healthcare professionals, educators, and families. This collaborative approach also helped us create a practical tool that could be applied in both clinical and educational contexts.

Our design process was iterative, meaning we continuously refined the questionnaire based on the feedback we received. We started with 85 items and carefully reduced them to a final set of 50. Our goal throughout this process was to ensure that the questions were clear, meaningful, and easy to understand for both children and their caregivers.

3.2 Contextual framework and practical relevance

The development of the PACOPED QL emerged from a broader vision to enhance PPC, grounded in the principles of patient-centered medicine and inclusive education. From the very beginning, our aim was not just to create a questionnaire—it was to inspire a cultural shift in how we understand and support the QoL of these children. We designed the PACOPED QL as a practical tool that healthcare professionals, educators, and caregivers can seamlessly integrate into their daily routines, enabling more personalized and meaningful interventions.

Thanks to its multidimensional design, the PACOPED QL can be adapted to various contexts, whether in hospitals, schools, or home settings. It allows us to evaluate essential aspects like social inclusion, access to educational activities, and the emotional impact of treatments. Importantly, the questionnaire moves beyond just assessing clinical status. It also considers how the child's social and educational environments influence their overall QoL, emphasizing the need for a holistic, whole-person approach.

3.3 Content validation: Commitment to multidisciplinary excellence

We validated the content of the PACOPED QL using the Delphi method, engaging 14 experts from diverse disciplines to ensure each item was evaluated from multiple perspectives. This collaborative approach allowed us to ensure that every question was not only relevant and understandable but also addressed critical aspects of children's well-being. Through several rounds of expert feedback, we refined the items to enhance their clarity and relevance. To ensure the quality of the questionnaire, we quantified the items using Aiken's V index, retaining only those with a score above 0.75. This meticulous process guaranteed that every question contributed meaningfully to a holistic evaluation of well-being. Our aim was to create a tool that offers a thorough and impactful assessment, aligned with the broader goal of supporting children in a comprehensive and meaningful way.

3.4 Pilot test: Grounded in feasibility and everyday realities

Once we completed the initial design of the PACOPED QL, we conducted a pilot test involving 40 children receiving palliative care and 81 of their primary caregivers. Our goal was not only to evaluate the consistency of the questionnaire items but also to understand how the tool could fit into the everyday lives of the participants. To achieve this, we used a dual-response design: children responded to the questions when possible, while caregivers provided complementary information. This approach allowed us to gather diverse perspectives, ensuring the inclusion of children with cognitive limitations. The results were promising, showing strong internal consistency, with Cronbach's alpha values exceeding 0.8 in most dimensions. This feedback helped us refine certain items, particularly those where inconsistencies or interpretive challenges arose. These adjustments focused on improving the user experience, making the questionnaire more intuitive and better suited for seamless use in various care settings.

3.5 Structural and psychometric validation: What is behind the numbers

To ensure the PACOPED QL was both reliable and meaningful, we conducted a structural and psychometric validation, going beyond simply checking if the questionnaire was consistent. One of the key steps was performing an exploratory factor analysis (EFA)—a statistical technique used to uncover the underlying structure of a set of questions. Essentially, EFA helps us confirm that the questions group together in a way that aligns with the dimensions we aimed to measure, like emotional well-being or social inclusion. To verify if our data was suitable for this analysis, we used two tests. Bartlett's test of sphericity checks whether there are relationships between the items—an essential condition for grouping them into meaningful factors. Meanwhile, the Kaiser-Meyer-Olkin (KMO) index measures how adequate the data is for factor analysis, with higher values indicating a better fit. In our case, the results showed a strong and coherent structure, confirming that the questionnaire works well as a whole.

But we did not stop at reliability. We also wanted to ensure the questionnaire could be used in different cultural contexts, given the diverse realities of PPC. To test this, we validated it with multicenter samples in Spain and Ecuador. This allowed us to see how participants from different backgrounds interpreted and responded to the questions. Analyses of internal consistency (which checks if the items within a dimension are closely related) and stability (which ensures responses remain reliable over time) showed that the questionnaire was not only reliable but also adaptable. This adaptability is critical in a field as complex and diverse as PPC, where the cultural and social contexts can significantly influence how QoL is perceived and supported. By making sure the PACOPED QL works across settings, we aimed to create a tool that truly reflects the experiences of children and their caregivers, no matter where they are.

3.6 Participants and sample: Embracing diversity and representativeness

Our study included 121 participants, comprising children in palliative care and their primary caregivers, recruited from specialized units in Spain and Ecuador. We used a purposive sampling method, which allowed us to include a diverse range of conditions and situations among children in palliative care. This approach was essential to ensure the questionnaire's applicability across a broad spectrum of cases. Involving caregivers as key participants was a deliberate choice, as they offer invaluable insights into the child's QoL while reflecting the perspectives of those most closely involved in daily care. This dual perspective—child and caregiver—was critical for capturing the child's overall experience and ensuring the instrument reflected the complexity of their realities.

3.7 Ethical considerations and social responsibility

Ethical integrity was at the heart of the PACOPED QL development process. In addition to following the guidelines established by the Declaration of Helsinki, we adhered to the principles of Open Science and Responsible Research and Innovation (RRI). These principles emphasize transparency, inclusivity, and accountability, guiding us to ensure the highest ethical standards. We took several measures to protect participant rights, including full anonymization of data and the use of clear, accessible informed consent forms for both caregivers and children. Our approach emphasized respecting the dignity and autonomy of every participant, making sure their involvement was both voluntary and meaningful.

3.8 Data analysis: Insights for action

We analyzed the collected data using R (version 4.1.2), employing both descriptive and inferential statistical techniques to delve deeply into the results. The Shapiro-Wilk test helped us assess whether the data followed a normal distribution, which is a foundational step in choosing appropriate statistical methods. When the data did not meet the assumptions of normality, we used non-parametric analyses to ensure the results remained rigorous and reliable.

Our analysis went beyond simply confirming the questionnaire's validity and reliability. We examined patterns that could inform future improvements and identified critical areas for intervention. For example, we explored group differences, such as variations in QoL across cultural contexts or disparities between caregiver and child perceptions. These findings not only validate the instrument but also highlight the need for interventions tailored to the unique realities of each patient and their environment, paving the way for further research and refinement of care practices.

3.9 Implications and future applications

The PACOPED QL is more than just a tool for measurement—it is a catalyst for intervention and decision-making. Its use in clinical, educational, and community settings opens up opportunities to plan personalized care, pinpoint areas that need improvement, and foster the social and educational inclusion of children in palliative care. The instrument's value goes far beyond simple assessment; it is designed to transform how we understand and support these children, serving as a guide for professionals and caregivers to actively enhance their QoL. This tool also has the potential to influence broader health and education policies. By generating reliable, relevant data about the QoL of children in palliative care, the PACOPED QL can support the development of initiatives that promote best practices in PPC. Additionally, it can help advocate for equitable access to tailored educational resources, ensuring that all children, regardless of their circumstances, receive the support they need to thrive. In this way, the PACOPED QL not only assesses the present but also shapes a more inclusive and compassionate future for children in palliative care and their families.

4. Dimensions of QoL in the PACOPED QL instrument

The PACOPED QL is built around eight key areas that together paint a full picture of what QoL means for children in palliative care. Based on Schalock and Verdugo's model [21], these areas are all connected, showing that each part of a child's well-being affects and is affected by the others. Here is an overview of each dimension and why it matters:

4.1 Physical well-being

Physical well-being is at the heart of understanding QoL, especially for children with chronic illnesses or those in palliative care. This dimension looks at things like pain, energy levels, and how much the child can take part in everyday activities. Managing pain and other symptoms effectively is essential in palliative care, as it helps children experience moments of comfort and joy, even in small ways. In the PACOPED QL, we focus on this area to ensure that care is not just about extending life but about making sure each day is as comfortable and dignified as possible.

4.2 Emotional well-being

Emotional well-being focuses on how children feel on the inside, including emotions like fear, sadness, and anxiety, as well as positive feelings like joy and hope. In palliative care, understanding these emotions is vital—not just to address pain or worry, but also to find sources of strength and happiness. By assessing this dimension, we can better understand how children cope with their illness and create personalized strategies to support their emotional stability and resilience.

4.3 Interpersonal relationships

Relationships are at the core of a child's life, especially when they face a serious illness. This dimension looks at how connected children feel to their family, friends, and caregivers. These interactions play a huge role in providing emotional safety and a sense of belonging. For children in palliative care, supportive relationships can be a powerful source of comfort and strength. Through this dimension, we aim to identify ways to strengthen these bonds, ensuring children feel accompanied and understood.

4.4 Social inclusion

Social inclusion is about making sure children feel part of their community and everyday activities, like school or play. Many children in palliative care face barriers that isolate them, which can impact their confidence and sense of belonging. This dimension evaluates how much the child is involved and treated as a valued member of society. By addressing challenges to inclusion, we can create opportunities for meaningful participation, enhancing their QoL.

4.5 Self-determination

Self-determination is the child's ability to make choices about their life, even in small ways. While their condition might limit their independence, being involved in decisions—whether about their care, daily activities, or preferences—helps them feel valued and in control. This dimension measures how much children feel they can express their wishes and have a say in their lives, boosting their confidence and sense of autonomy.

4.6 Rights

Every child has basic rights, like being treated with respect, receiving proper care, and having their voice heard. This dimension focuses on whether these rights are upheld, ensuring children are treated with the dignity they deserve. In palliative care, respecting these rights is not just ethical—it directly enhances their well-being and sense of worth.

4.7 Material well-being

Material well-being looks at whether children and their families have access to the resources they need, like a safe home, proper food, and financial support for medical or daily necessities. For families dealing with a life-limiting illness, these resources can make a big difference in how they cope. This dimension helps identify any gaps and ensures that children have a stable and supportive environment.

4.8 Personal development

Personal development is about giving children opportunities to learn, grow, and explore their interests, even when facing severe illness. This dimension looks at whether children can continue to develop their skills and achieve personal milestones, no matter how small. These opportunities allow them to maintain a sense of purpose and progress, contributing to their overall well-being and happiness.

5. Why multidimensionality matters today

The multidimensional approach of the PACOPED QL provides a deep and well-rounded view of the well-being of children in palliative care. Each dimension sheds light on a different aspect of the child's life, and together, they create a complete picture that allows for more personalized and meaningful interventions. In today's world, where pediatric care increasingly focuses on integration and putting the patient at the center, an instrument like this—addressing physical, emotional, social, and personal growth—ensures that care truly prioritizes QoL in all its forms. The PACOPED QL is designed not just to measure but to *inspire action*. By highlighting specific areas that need attention, it empowers professionals and caregivers to make meaningful changes that directly improve the child's life. It transforms assessment into practical steps, helping children live fuller, more meaningful lives, even in the face of complex challenges.

6. How the PACOPED QL makes a difference in everyday care

The PACOPED QL was created to be a practical tool that works in the real-world settings where children in palliative care live, learn, and grow. Whether it is in hospitals, schools, or community programs, this tool helps professionals understand what each child needs to improve their QoL. Here is how it is used and why it is important for bringing different areas of care together (**Table 1**).

In healthcare settings, the PACOPED QL is a vital tool for looking beyond medical treatments to the broader needs of the child. It helps doctors, nurses, and other health professionals understand how pain, emotional well-being, and other factors impact the child's overall QoL. The results guide personalized care plans that prioritize comfort and dignity while addressing physical and emotional challenges. For instance, if the questionnaire reveals unaddressed pain or high anxiety, healthcare providers can adjust treatment strategies to improve the child's comfort and engagement in daily life. This holistic view ensures that care decisions support not just survival but also meaningful, positive experiences for the child.

In schools, the PACOPED QL helps educators understand the unique barriers that children in palliative care may face, such as difficulties with inclusion, participation, or developmental progress. Armed with this knowledge, teachers can adapt the classroom environment and learning strategies to better meet the child's needs. This might involve tailoring lesson plans, creating flexible schedules, or providing additional support to ensure the child feels included and engaged. By fostering cognitive and emotional growth in a supportive setting, educators can help these children stay connected to their peers and continue to learn despite their health challenges.

In the broader community, the PACOPED QL serves as a guide for organizations that provide support to children with complex illnesses and their families. The questionnaire identifies areas where families may need more help, such as access to in-home care, inclusive recreational activities, or additional financial support. Community programs can use this data to develop services that complement efforts

Applications	Highlights
Clinical	• Vital tool for holistic care in healthcare settings. • Guides personalized care plans addressing pain, emotional well-being, and QoL. • Adjusts treatment strategies for better comfort and meaningful experiences.
Educational	• Identifies barriers to inclusion and participation in schools. • Helps adapt classroom environments and learning strategies. • Supports cognitive and emotional growth in a tailored, inclusive setting.
Community	• Highlights family support needs, such as in-home care or financial aid. • Guides community programs to complement healthcare and education efforts. • Promotes comprehensive care, including inclusive recreational activities.
Multidisciplinary collaboration	• Encourages coordination among health care, education, and community professionals. • Integrates expertise to address physical, emotional, and social needs. • Ensures a cohesive approach to the child's well-being.
Public policy	• Provides data to identify gaps in health care, education, and social support. • Advocates for better resources, inclusive initiatives, and financial aid. • Supports evidence-based policy changes to foster inclusivity and compassion.

Table 1.
Highlights of PACOPED QL applications.

in health care and education, ensuring that all aspects of the child's life are supported. For example, a recreational program designed to promote social inclusion can work hand-in-hand with clinical pain management and educational adaptations, creating a more comprehensive care framework.

The true strength of the PACOPED QL lies in its ability to bring together professionals from different disciplines. Physicians, nurses, psychologists, social workers, teachers, and community volunteers can all use the insights from the questionnaire to address various aspects of the child's well-being. For example, healthcare providers may address physical symptoms highlighted in the questionnaire, while psychologists focus on emotional well-being, and educators adjust the school environment to enhance inclusion. This shared understanding encourages collaboration, ensuring that all facets of the child's life are cared for in a coordinated way, with each professional contributing their expertise.

The PACOPED QL does not just benefit individual children—it has the potential to shape public policies. By providing clear and reliable data on the QoL of children in palliative care, the questionnaire highlights gaps and opportunities in health care, education, and social support systems. Policymakers can use this information to advocate for better resources and programs, such as specialized training for healthcare professionals, inclusive education initiatives, or financial support for families. For example, national guidelines for PPC could be informed by data from the PACOPED QL, ensuring that every child receives equitable and comprehensive support. This evidence-based approach helps build awareness, drive investment, and create policies that improve the lives of children with complex medical needs and their families, fostering a more inclusive and compassionate society.

While the PACOPED QL also holds potential for influencing public policy in health care and education, we recognize that this is an ambitious goal. Changing policy is a complex process, but this instrument represents an important first step by providing the evidence and insights needed to advocate for meaningful systemic change. Even small advancements in awareness and resource allocation can make a significant difference over time.

The PACOPED QL is more than just a tool for measuring QoL—it is a practical resource for driving meaningful interventions. Its multidimensional design and emphasis on real-world usability not only allow us to assess the well-being of children in palliative care but also inspire concrete improvements in the way care is delivered. What makes the PACOPED QL especially relevant is its ability to bring together all the key people in a child's life—healthcare professionals, educators, and community members—offering a shared framework to actively enhance the QoL for these children and their families.

7. Building on the PACOPED QL: Challenges and next steps

While the PACOPED QL has made a significant impact in understanding and supporting the QoL of children in palliative care, there are still challenges to overcome and opportunities for growth. Addressing these will help ensure the tool reaches its full potential and continues to make a difference in the lives of children, families, and professionals.

One major challenge is adapting the questionnaire to diverse cultural and socioeconomic contexts. Healthcare and education systems vary widely across countries, and for the PACOPED QL to be truly effective, it must be flexible and culturally sensitive. This requires more than translation—it involves tailoring the questionnaire to reflect local cultural norms, values, and conditions. Cross-cultural validation will be key to ensuring the instrument remains accurate and relevant, no matter the setting.

Another hurdle lies in integrating the PACOPED QL into the daily workflows of professionals. Even though the tool is designed to be practical, limited resources and heavy workloads in some settings may create barriers to its use. Overcoming this requires strategies to train professionals effectively and to streamline the implementation process. Future developments could include embedding the PACOPED QL into electronic medical record systems or creating automated tools for data collection and analysis, reducing the administrative burden on already stretched teams. Research should also explore how the PACOPED QL can evaluate the impact of specific interventions on children's QoL. For example, studies could investigate how well the tool measures the effectiveness of personalized educational programs, innovative pain management techniques, or psychosocial support systems. These insights would not only refine the tool further but also provide evidence-based recommendations for broader adoption of successful strategies in diverse contexts.

Digitalizing the PACOPED QL represents another promising direction for enhancing its accessibility and usability. Developing mobile apps or online platforms could simplify data collection, allow for real-time monitoring, and provide quicker, more precise feedback. Digital versions could also make the questionnaire more engaging and interactive for children, especially those with communication or cognitive challenges, by incorporating visuals or adaptive technologies. Additionally, digital tools could empower caregivers and professionals with immediate insights, enabling timely and targeted interventions.

By addressing these challenges and pursuing these directions, the PACOPED QL can continue to evolve as a powerful, transformative tool—not just for assessing QoL, but for actively improving it for children in palliative care and those who support them.

8. A step toward transforming care: Conclusions

The PACOPED QL marks a meaningful shift in PPC, offering a deeply human and comprehensive approach to understanding the QoL of children with life-limiting conditions. This tool goes far beyond simply measuring well-being; it serves as a call to action for all those involved in the care of these children. It reminds us to look beyond medical symptoms and see the child as a whole person, with emotional, social, educational, and personal dimensions that deserve attention and care.

In a world where health care can sometimes feel impersonal or overly technical, the PACOPED QL emphasizes the importance of compassion and connection. It challenges us to not only prolong life but to make every moment meaningful, comfortable, and dignified. By placing the child and their family at the center, this tool fosters a collaborative approach where physicians, nurses, psychologists, educators, caregivers, and communities work together to create a more holistic and nurturing care system. While the path forward is not without challenges, the PACOPED QL offers a vision of what is possible. It illuminates the potential for truly inclusive and compassionate care that adapts to the unique needs of each child. Its ultimate measure of success will not lie in the numbers it generates but in the tangible changes it inspires—helping caregivers feel more supported, professionals feel more empowered, and, most importantly, children feel seen, valued, and loved.

The challenges we face in adapting the PACOPED QL to diverse cultural and practical contexts are real. Yet, this tool lays the foundation for continued innovation and progress. It is a first step in building systems of care that listen to children and their families, recognize their voices, and honor their experiences. Through this work, we aspire to create a world where every child, regardless of their condition, can live a life filled with meaning and connection. The PACOPED QL is a reminder that even in the face of great challenges, there is always room for dignity, compassion, and hope—and that these qualities can transform care into something truly life-affirming.

Acknowledgements

We thank the children and families who participated in this study, as well as the multidisciplinary team of professionals whose expertise was vital to the development of the PACOPED QL. We also acknowledge the institutions in Spain and Ecuador that supported this work and the funding agencies that made it possible. This work was supported by the Ministry of science and innovation of Spain [PID2020-114712RB-I00], and the corresponding author is funded by the Spanish National Research Agency (MCIN/AEI/10.13039/501100011033) and the European Social Fund Plus (ESF+) (PRE2021-097050). Finally, we are grateful to our reviewers and collaborators for their invaluable feedback.

Author details

Laia Riera-Negre*, Maria Rosa Rosselló and Sebastià Verger
University of the Balearic Islands, Palma, Spain

*Address all correspondence to: laia.riera@uib.cat

References

[1] Avendaño MJ, Barra E. Autoeficacia, apoyo social y calidad de vida en adolescentes con enfermedades crónicas. Terapia Psicológica. 2008;**26**(2):165-172. DOI: 10.4067/S0718-48082008000200002

[2] Jaimes-Valencia ML, Fajardo-Nates S, Arguello JF, Mejía-Arciniegas CN, Rojas-Arenas LC, Gallo-Eugenio LM, et al. Percepciones de padres o acudientes sobre la salud y calidad de vida de sus hijos adolescentes escolarizados. MedUNAB. 2018;**21**(3):314-333. DOI: 10.29375/01237047.2736

[3] Sheng N, Ma J, Ding W, Zhang Y. Effects of caregiver-involved interventions on the quality of life of children and adolescents with chronic conditions and their caregivers: A systematic review and meta-analysis. Quality of Life Research. 2019;**28**:13-33. DOI: 10.1007/s11136-018-1976-3

[4] Varni JW, Limbers CA, Burwinkle TM. Impaired health-related quality of life in children and adolescents with chronic conditions: A comparative analysis of 10 disease clusters and 33 disease categories/severities utilizing the PedsQL™ 4.0 Generic Core Scales. Health and Quality of Life Outcomes. 2007;**5**:1-15. DOI: 10.1186/1477-7525-5-43

[5] World Health Organization. Measuring Quality of Life: The World Health Organization Quality of Life Instruments (WHOQOL-100 and WHOQOL-BREF). Geneva: World Health Organization; 2012. Available from: https://www.who.int/tools/whoqol

[6] Bergstraesser E. Pediatric palliative care—When quality of life becomes the main focus of treatment. European Journal of Pediatrics. 2013;**172**(2):139-150. DOI: 10.1007/s00431-012-1710-z

[7] Himelstein BP, Hilden JM, Boldt AM, Weissman D. Pediatric palliative care. The New England Journal of Medicine. 2004;**350**(17):1752-1762. DOI: 10.1056/NEJMra030334

[8] Kittelsen TB, Lorentsen VB, Castor C, Lee A, Kvarme LG, Winger A. It's about living a normal life: Parents' quality of life when their child has a life-threatening or life-limiting condition-a qualitative study. BMC Palliative Care. 2024;**23**(1):92. DOI: 10.1186/s12904-024-01417-3

[9] Sisk BA, Feudtner C, Bluebond-Langner M, Sourkes B, Hinds PS, Wolfe J. Response to suffering of the seriously ill child: A history of palliative care for children. Pediatrics. 2020;**145**(1):e20191741. DOI: 10.1542/peds.2019-1741

[10] Wallner M, Haselmayer D, Nagl-Cupal M, Eppel-Meichlinger J, Mayer H. Building a programme theory of a specialist paediatric palliative and hospice care programme: Development process and methodological reflection. BMC Palliative Care. 2024;**23**(1):180. DOI: 10.1186/s12904-024-01492-6

[11] European Association for Palliative Care. IMPaCCT: Standards for paediatric palliative care in Europe. European Journal of Palliative Care. 2007;**14**(3):109-114. Available from: https://www.redpal.es/wp-content/uploads/2018/12/IMPaCCTSp.-estandares-CPP-Europa.pdf

[12] Toro-Pérez D, Limonero JT, Guillen M, Bolancé C, Vilarrubí SN, Camprodon-Rosanas E. Evaluating

quality of life in pediatric palliative care: A cross-sectional analysis of children's and parents' perspectives. European Journal of Pediatrics. 2024;**183**(3):1305-1314. DOI: 10.1007/s00431-023-05330-4

[13] Dombrecht L, Lacerda A, Wolfe J, Snaman J. A call to improve pediatric palliative care quality through research. BMC Palliative Care. 2023;**22**(1):12. DOI: 10.1186/s12904-023-01262-w

[14] Ruiz-Gil T, Ródenas-Rigla F. Quality of care in pediatric palliative care: A scoping review. Children. 2023;**10**(12):1922. DOI: 10.3390/children10121922

[15] Compas BE, Jaser SS, Dunn MJ, Rodriguez EM. Coping with chronic illness in childhood and adolescence. Annual Review of Clinical Psychology. 2012;**8**:455-480. DOI: 10.1146/annurev-clinpsy-032511-143108

[16] Eiser C, Morse R. The measurement of quality of life in children: Past and future perspectives. Journal of Developmental and Behavioral Pediatrics. 2001;**22**(4):248-256. DOI: 10.1097/00004703-200108000-00007

[17] Reilly C, Agnew R, Neville BGR. Depression and anxiety in childhood epilepsy: A review. Seizure. 2011;**20**(8):589-597. DOI: 10.1016/j.seizure.2011.06.004

[18] Ainscow M, Booth T, Dyson A. Improving Schools, Developing Inclusion. London: Routledge; 2006. DOI: 10.4324/9780203967157

[19] Robinson S, Summers K. An evaluation of the educational support for teachers who teach children with life limiting illness in schools. Pastoral Care in Education. 2012;**30**(3):191-207. DOI: 10.1080/02643944.2012.671341

[20] UNICEF. Inclusive Education: Ensuring every Child Learns. Geneva: UNICEF; 2020. Available from: https://www.unicef.org/education/inclusive-education

[21] Schalock RL, Verdugo MÁ. El Concepto de Calidad de Vida en los Servicios y Apoyos para Personas con Discapacidad Intelectual. 2007. Available from: https://hdl.handle.net/20.500.12365/18060

[22] Riera-Negre L, Varona J, Rosselló MR, Verger S. PACOPED QL: Development and evaluation of the quality-of-life scale for children with life-threatening illnesses. Palliative and Supportive Care. 2025;**23**:e19. DOI: 10.1017/S1478951524001779

[23] Schalock RL, Verdugo MA, Gomez LE, Reinders HS. Moving us toward a theory of individual quality of life. American Journal on Intellectual and Developmental Disabilities. 2016;**121**(1):1-12. DOI: 10.1352/1944-7558-121.1.1

[24] Eiser C, Morse R. A review of measures of quality of life for children with chronic illness. Archives of Disease in Childhood. 2001;**84**(3):205-211. DOI: 10.1136/adc.84.3.205

[25] Palermo TM, Long AC, Lewandowski AS, Drotar D, Quittner AL, Walker LS. Evidence-based assessment of health-related quality of life and functional impairment in pediatric psychology. Journal of Pediatric Psychology. 2008;**33**(9):983-996. DOI: 10.1093/jpepsy/jsn038

[26] Umaretiya PJ, Wolfe J. Achieving global pediatric palliative care equity—What we have yet to learn. JAMA Network Open. 2022;**5**(3):e221253. DOI: 10.1001/jamanetworkopen.2022.1253

[27] Papa S, Mercante A, Giacomelli L, Benini F. Pediatric palliative care: Insights into assessment tools and review instruments. Children. 2023;**10**(8):1406. DOI: 10.3390/children10081406

[28] Jiang S, Wang L, Jiang C, Tan S. Effects of multidimensional social exclusion on child well-being: An examination of migration paradox in Chinese children. Journal of Child and Family Studies. 2024;**33**(1):39-52. DOI: 10.1007/s10826-023-02606-z

[29] Avoine-Blondin J, Parent V, Fasse L, Lopez C, Humbert N, Duval M, et al. How do professionals assess the quality of life of children with advanced cancer receiving palliative care, and what are their recommendations for improvement? BMC Palliative Care. 2018;**17**:71. DOI: 10.1186/s12904-018-0328-y

Chapter 7

Evaluation of Practices and Management of Pain in Children at the Mother and Child Centre of the Chantal Biya Foundation

Angèle Hermine Pondy Ongotsoyi,
Laura Murielle Kuate Makowa, Patience Tazanou Ngouanet,
Louise Loe Renee and Audrey Miyehane

Abstract

Pain in Cameroonian society is not always considered a health problem; enduring pain is a sign of courage. The objective of our study was to evaluate the knowledge, attitudes and practices of CME/FCB physicians on pain in children and its management. A descriptive and analytical CAP study was conducted at the CME/FCB from June 2020 to January 2021. We compared the physician survey with patient records seen during the same time. Fifty doctors were included, and 200 hospitalisation records were analysed. The average number of years of service was 4.28 ± 3.81 years. The knowledge of pain assessment was 20% good, moderate 64%, and 16% insufficient. Among doctors, 50% say they systematically assess pain. In the review of the 200 records, pain was assessed in 4 cases, or 4% by the Visual Analogue Scale 60%. The quality of attitudes was approximately 44%, 30% wrong, and 26% fair. Painful medical procedures were performed in 62 (31%) of the cases during the study period, and 92% of these patients had not received premedication. Hospital physicians had a lack of knowledge and there was underestimation and insufficient management of pain in children's charts.

Keywords: pain, child, evaluation, scales, symptoms

1. Introduction

Pain is an unpleasant stimulus, occurring as a result of injury, illness or medical procedures experienced by adults and children, including newborns [1]. It is associated with increased anxiety, avoidance, somatic disorders and increased distress of parents [2]. Pain is felt at any age, according to the American Medical Association; infants and children experience painful stimuli more intensely than adults, due to the inflammatory response and the absence of central inhibitory influence [3]. Infants and children, who experience pain early in life, have been shown to show long-term

IntechOpen

changes in their perception of pain, eating and sleep disorders [4]. In Cameroonian socio-cultural representation, pain is not always seen as a health problem, and enduring pain is proof of courage. Pain management is not a major concern; personal beliefs, lack of training, and insufficient devices and medications are the factors that can influence the management of the child's pain. The literature is full of tools for pain assessment and management [1, 5, 6]. As pain is a real concern in paediatrics with harmful consequences if not treated, we conducted a study, so the objective was to evaluate the knowledge, attitudes and practices of the doctors of the Mother and Child Centre of the Chantal Biya Foundation (CME/FCB) on the pain of the child and its management.

2. Methodology

We conducted a descriptive and analytical study of the Knowledge, Attitude, Practice (CAP) type at the Mother and Child Centre of the Chantal Biya Foundation of Yaoundé (CME-FCB). A reference university paediatric hospital in Cameroon, which has emergency, nephrology, neurology, endocrinology, cardiology, infectiology, resuscitation, neonatology, nutrition, haematology and paediatric oncology services from June 2020 to January 2021.

The study population consisted of the emergency department physicians, the physicians taking night shift at the emergency room, the paediatricians supervising the emergency room, and the records of the 0–14-year-olds examined during the study period.

Our work was divided into two parts:

- The first part was the inclusion of doctors through the filling in of an individual technical sheet that allowed them to evaluate their knowledge, and determine their attitudes and practices on the evaluation and management of pain in children.

- The second part consisted of checking the practices of each doctor from the study of the patient records seen by the various doctors included in the study.

Ethical considerations: the administrative authorisation was given by the Mother and Child Centre of the Chantal Biya Foundation. Consent forms were signed by the participants. These consents indicated the purpose of the study and the benefits. Participation was voluntary.

Questionnaire: Two structured questionnaires were designed. The first was administered to the participants to obtain demographic information (8 questions), knowledge on the evaluation of the child's pain (6 questions), attitude of the doctors toward the child's pain (7 questions), and practice for the management of the child's pain (11 questions). The second questionnaire completed by the investigators comprised 8 questions evaluating the demographic information, pathologies, evaluation and management of the patient's pain seen by these doctors.

Statistical analysis: The full knowledge, attitude and practice scores were 20, 20 and 12, respectively. The scores of all the questions in each part had been summed to give the total score as a percentage-weighted index score for the level of knowledge, attitudes and practices in child pain assessment and management. According to the KAP study methodology, the overall knowledge assessment was rated as follows: 0–50%:

poor knowledge, 50–65%: insufficient knowledge, 65–85%: average knowledge, ˃85%: good knowledge. Assessment of overall attitudes: 0–50%: negative attitudes, 50–65%: wrong attitudes, 65–85%: approximate attitudes, ˃85%: right attitudes. Global Practice Assessment [7]: 0–50%: harmful practices, 50–70%: inadequate practices, ˃70: adequate practices. Quantitative data processing was carried out using Epi-Info version 3.5.4 and Microsoft Office Excel 2013 software. Continuous variables were summarised as means and standard deviations, and categorical variables were reported as frequencies and percentages for evaluation of descriptive statistics results. The odd ratios were calculated to assess risk factors. P value <0.05 was considered statistically significant.

3. Results

We included 50 doctors and analysed 200 patient records. The average age of the physicians was 33.08 ± 7.73 years. The sex ratio was 0.35. General Practitioners (GPs) were the most represented with a percentage of 42%, 12% were paediatricians, 26% were junior residents, and 20% were senior residents. Professional experience had a mean year of service of 4.28 ± 3.81 years, (34) 74% of physicians had experience of 5 years or less and (05) 10% had experience of more than 11 years, (08) 16% had experience of 6–10 years (**Figures 1–3**).

3.1 How well doctors know how to evaluate pain in children

During the surveys, screaming and crying were the signs known by the doctors (100%), while slowness, rarity of movements (16%), and an expressionless child (12%) were less known as signs referring to pain. Doctors thought the presence of parents was necessary to approach the painful child at 90%, and 94% thought that routine assessment of the child's pain at entry with a suitable scale would improve management. All physicians reported assessing pain in children they received in consultation, and the most well-known scales were: Visual Analogue Scale (VAS), Single Verbal Scale (SPE), Digital Scale (EN), Six Face Scale, 92% Male Scheme, 92, 70, 70,

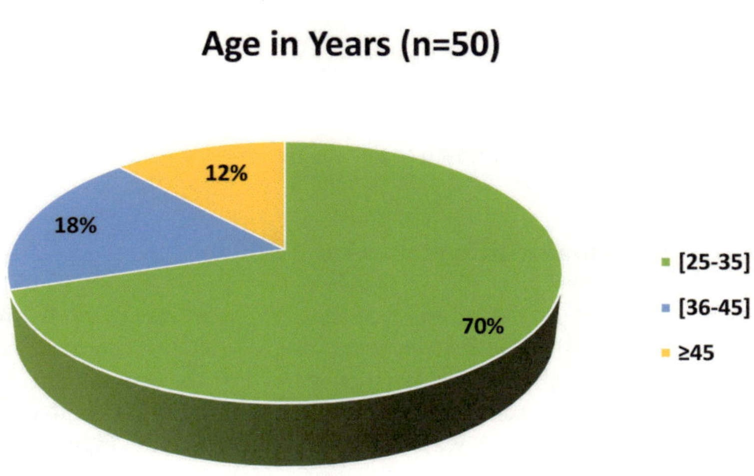

Figure 1.
Physician age.

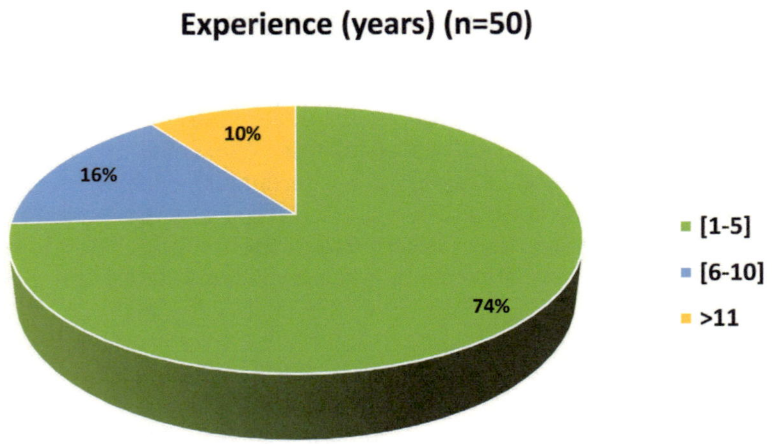

Figure 2.
Physician experience.

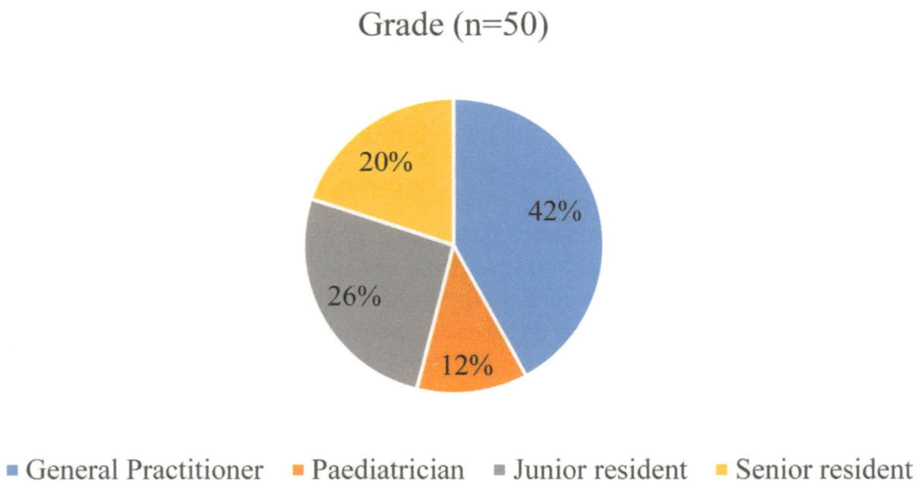

Figure 3.
Physician grade.

and 60%, respectively. The least known scale was the *comfort scale* with a percentage of 2% (**Figure 4**).

3.2 Physician attitudes toward pain evaluation

In our study, (18) 9% of physicians reported assessing pain "rarely" in children they received in consultation, while (14) 28% reported "often," (11) 22% reported "occasionally," and (16) 8% reported "always." Upon patient entry into the centre, (6) 12% reported assessing pain while (19) 38% assessed pain during hospitalisation and (25) 50% assessed pain systematically. A validated scale was used in 20% of physicians (**Figure 5**).

Six out of 10 physicians, or 60%, used the visual analogue scale as a pain rating scale, while 40% used the simple verbal scale. Barriers to pain assessment were

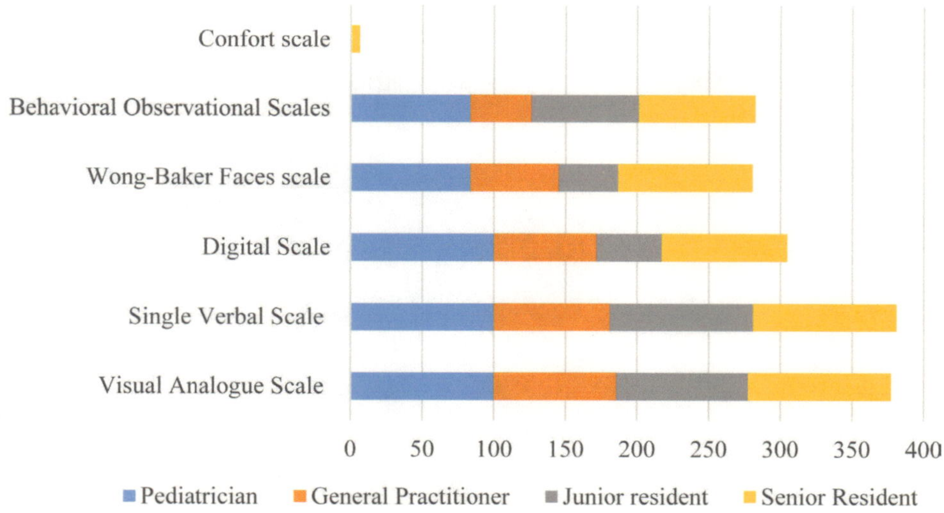

Figure 4.
Knowledge of pain assessment scales by grade.

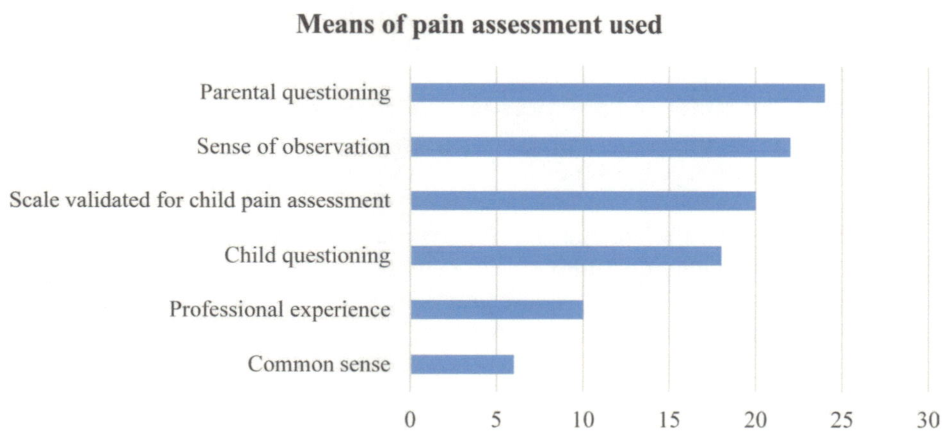

Figure 5.
How doctors evaluate pain.

communication with the child (54%), non-adherence of the child (46%), lack of rating scale (38%), lack of time (36%), and forgetting (2%) (**Figure 6**).

3.3 Physician practices

Doctors (45) 90% did not have a pain management protocol in their departments. For pharmacological management, the drugs used were paracetamol 100%, tramadol 92%, non-steroidal anti-inflammatory drugs 86%, morphine injectable 30%, and paracetamol codeine 20%.

Non-pharmacological measures used were breastfeeding (86%), distraction (64%), massage (58%), and non-nutritive sucking (36%).

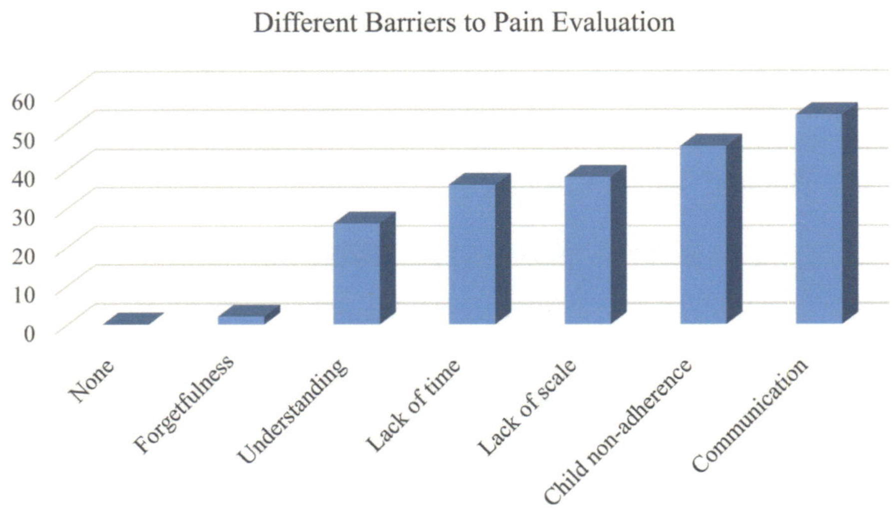

Figure 6.
Different barriers to pain evaluation.

In the face of pain, 48% did not use pain management methods, 16% used xylocaine, 8% used EMLA cream and 12% used distraction.

3.4 Knowledge, attitudes and practices assessment score

Knowledge was average in (32) 64%, (8) 16% were inadequate, and (10) 20% were well known.

For attitudes, (22) 44% had approximate attitudes (13) 26% of negative attitudes and (15) 30% of erroneous attitudes.

For practices, (24) 48% had adequate practices, (24) 48% were inadequate, and (2) only 4% had harmful practices (**Figure 7**).

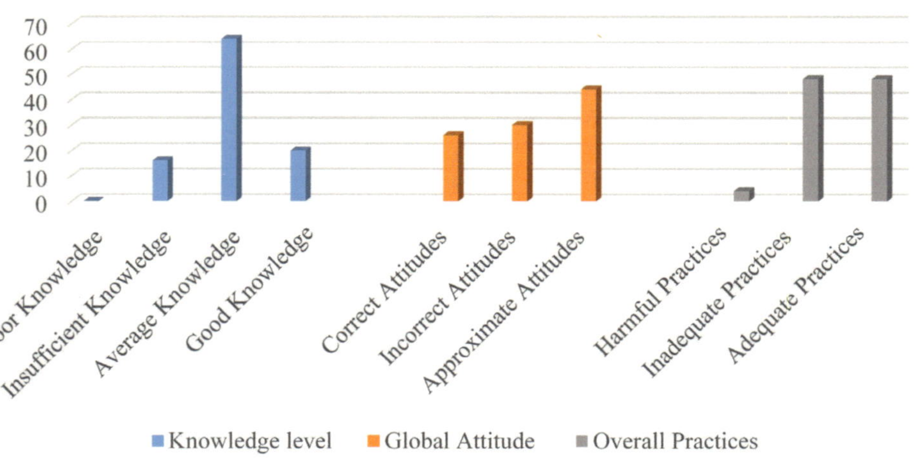

Figure 7.
Physician knowledge, attitudes and practice on child pain.

Variables	Inadequate practices			OR (IC 95%)	P value
	Yes n (%)	No n(%)	Total n(%)		
Wrong attitudes					
Yes	27 (58.7)	19 (41.3)	46 (92)	—	**0.040**
No	0 (0)	4 (100)	4 (8)		

Table 1.
Relationship between incorrect attitudes and inadequate practices.

3.4.1 Search for association factors

No significant relationship was found between gender, age, grade, seniority and insufficient knowledge. However, seniority ≥11 years was protective of erroneous attitudes with an odd ratio of 0.03 (0–0.65) and a P value = 0.020. Also, the paediatric grade was protective at 0.05 (0–0.82) and a P value of 0.030 for erroneous attitudes and inappropriate practices with an odd ratio of 0 (0–0.47) and a P value of 0.010.

No significant link was found between inadequate knowledge and mistaken attitudes, nor between inadequate knowledge and inadequate practices (**Table 1**).

There is a significant relationship between wrong attitudes and inappropriate practices with a P value of 0.04. 58% of our sample had wrong attitudes and inappropriate practices. Insufficient knowledge exposed 1.03 (0.26–4.24) times to improper practices. In our study, 6 of the 50 physicians surveyed had inadequate knowledge and practices.

4. File review

The mean age of our patients was 66.3 ± 45.3 with a minimum of 06 months and a maximum of 168 months, i.e., 14 years. A sex ratio of 1.4. The pain assessment of the

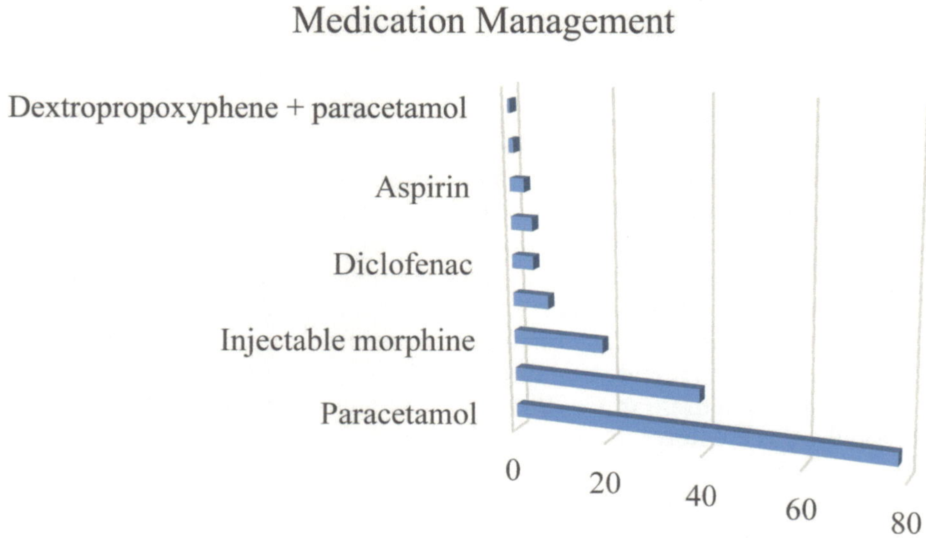

Figure 8.
Drug management of pain.

200 files collected was performed in only 09 files, i.e., 4.5%, and the rating scale used was the visual analogue scale. A medical procedure that could cause pain was performed on 62 patients, or 31.0%. Myelogram was 61.3%, lumbar puncture was 27%, and other procedures were 11.7%. Pain management prerequisites were found in only 13 cases in our sample, 6.5% primarily by xylocaine. Non-drug management of pain was found in 04 patients, including breastfeeding and massage. The most commonly used analgesics were paracetamol (78%), tramadol (39%) morphine for injection (19%) (**Figure 8**).

5. Discussion

5.1 Characteristics of our study population

5.1.1 Physician population: Age, length of service and grade

Pain in children is a reality and underestimated in our context [8]. Many childhood illnesses are accompanied by pain from common acute diseases such as angina, urinary tract infections, malaria, etc., to chronic diseases such as homozygous sickle cell disease in our context [9–11]. Pain is a perception that differs depending on the child's age [12, 13]. Recognition of pain and its evaluation will depend on the desire to search for pain and the skills of health professionals [14]. In our study, the mean age of the doctors was 33.08 years, with the extremes of 25 and 45 years with a sex ratio of 0.35. Freitas et al. in a study of child pain also found a predominance of females [8]. General practitioners accounted for 42% with professional experience between 1 and 15 years and an average of 4.28 ± 3.81 years. These data are similar to Kim et al. data in Korea, which had an average physician age of 29.9 years and an average duration of practice of 2.7 years [15].

5.1.2 Knowledge of pain assessment

Our population studied was a minimum of 06 months and a maximum of 168 months, or 14 years of age. In paediatrics, the expression of pain depends on age [12]. Thus, the newborn and the infant perceive pain but do not express it like the older child and the adolescent. The symptoms and clinical signs of pain as well as the pain assessment tools depend on the age and cognitive development of children [5]. In our study, screaming and crying were known as signs of pain; alone they refer to other perceptions in newborns and infants, such as hunger, sweating, and cold. Considering crying and screaming as referring to pain in this age group is not enough; they must be associated with other conditions such as the inability to calm the child, insomnia, reactions such as agitated movements, slowness, and a scarcity of movements. Expressing pain at this age is made difficult by the impossibility of using speech. Psychomotor atony, an extreme sign of pain, is found in a child who has lost all interest in those around him due to prolonged pain. The child becomes expressionless, as if empty with a smooth face, with no response from him when asked.

This is a serious sign that requires urgent diagnosis and treatment [16]. These findings were not found in our study and were due to a lack of knowledge of signs of pain in infants. In children aged 2 to 7 years, signs such as fear, anxiety, or aggression refer to pain, but this component of pain in children is often overlooked [17]. This lack of knowledge leads to an underestimation of the child's pain; in fact, Vincent et al. found that children are not always believed by their families and carers in their expression of pain because they are sometimes seen as exaggerating their pain [18]. Thus, there is a lack of knowledge of the child's signs of pain. Linhares et al. show in their study that 68% of the children interviewed claimed to have pain, but only 38% of the doctors found pain [19, 20]. Pain assessment makes it possible to render a subjective phenomenon objective, and thus, by using valid objective tools, it is possible to confirm the existence of pain, assess the intensity, determine the necessary analgesic means, to evaluate the effectiveness of the instituted treatment, and to adapt the treatment. Thus, good training in recognising pain in children and using valid age-appropriate tools will lead to good pain management [5].

The need for parents to be present at the child's visit was recognised in 90% of doctors, who said their presence was necessary to address the painful child. Subhashini et al. found the same notion in 93.5% of the staff studied [2].

Indeed, the presence of the parent with their sick child is necessary, especially if it is an infant, a young child or even an older child. Good communication between the parents of the sick child and the health professional aims to put the child at ease and create familiar contact with him, even if this objective is not easy to achieve from the first contact. On the other hand, this parental presence does not condition the assessment of the child's pain, which represents a professional technique for better care.

Some parents could reassure children and explain the treatment in familiar terms to them, especially during procedures such as lumbar, bone marrow, or pleural punctures; a good understanding of the parents and their adherence to the procedure makes it easier to carry out and generates fewer fears from children [21]. Assessing the child's pain is a challenge, a daily task that is truly carried out from the first visit and throughout their hospital stay. It requires being able to remain in an essential relationship, have a score, and adapt therapies. Whether it is an acute pain illness-related or chronic pain, the presence of parents is not necessary to affirm and assess the child's pain. All doctors in our study assessed pain in the children they saw for consultation, and 94% reported that routine pain assessment at entry by an appropriate scale improves pain management.

Pain assessment only at entry or during consultation is insufficient. The pain may get worse or less over time. The first treatment, therefore, requires an evaluation throughout the child's stay and would make it possible to modify the treatment. This attitude indicates a lack of adequate pain management for children by health professionals.

The best-known scales were 92% Visual Analogue Scale (VAS), 92% Verbal Simple Scale (VSS), and 70% numerical Scale (NS). In our study, physicians had little knowledge of the hetero-assessment tools that are needed to assess pain in infants and young children. The best-known self-assessment scale (VSS) in our study population is the least mentioned in practice. The best use scale in practice is visual analogue Scale (VAS), which is not familiar to our physicians; the reason is unknown. Nevertheless, we can highlight the absence of assessment tools in the services as a barrier to knowledge and assessment of pain with this scale. These data are better than those found by Freitas et al., which had only 31.1% knowledge of scales and 8.8% use [8]. Mentioning knowledge of the tools does not mean use appropriate to the child's age and/or disability. In our study, the use of EVS by all healthcare professionals reflects the lack of accurate data on signs and symptoms of pain across age groups.

5.1.3 Physician attitudes toward pain evaluation

Our study found that only 20% of doctors used valid scales, while 80% used subjective methods to assess pain. Therefore, among the barriers to pain assessment mentioned, only the lack of tools can be considered. Other reasons cannot be considered barriers because the hetero assessment that is done by healthcare practitioners using multiple items does not require patient participation for evaluation.

We found a discrepancy between the responses from the survey of health professionals and their handling of the files reviewed by them. Only 4.5% of these cases were assessed on a scale. These scales were not appropriate for the child's age and situation and could not allow for team-to-team monitoring. Moreover, only 8% of the doctors interviewed said that they "always" evaluated pain in children they received in consultation, while 28% evaluated it "often," 22% "occasionally," and 9% "rarely." Yet pain must be evaluated throughout the disease because pain treatment must be offered at the same time as the causative treatment. The study by Bougtoub et al. in 2012 found a systematic evaluation of 17% [22]. Stevens et al. in Canada found that in a population of 2987 children, pain was managed in only 28.3% of documented painful procedures [23]. Yet the stress and discomfort associated with pain have long-term negative effects on patients and their parents/carers. It can contribute to eating and sleeping disorders, cause post-traumatic stress disorder, decrease social skills, or increase fears [4]. In our study, for the management of pain caused by a painful gesture, only 6% of children had premedication, the main one being injectable xylocaine, which is also a source of pain and crying in children. This result indicates that premedication of painful procedures is not considered in our context; 90% of the doctors concerned declare that they do not have a protocol for managing the pain induced in their departments.

5.1.4 Physician practices

The survey of professionals shows that the practitioners' assertions are erroneous, and we can therefore conclude that pain management is not effective in the health facility. The shortcomings of health professionals are explained in this study by the different obstacles observed, which were communication, non-compliance of the child, lack of scale, lack of time, understanding and forgetting.

Inadequate scale leads to misinterpretation of pain and inadequate management. Pain evaluation is the first step in successful pain management [24]. Carers' attitude to the child's pain differs from what is known. Indeed, as Kim et al. point out, while many doctors believe they are highly trained in managing pain, they have insufficient attitudes and a level of knowledge [15]. Assessing and understanding what the child may be experiencing requires empathy for the child and family, observation of the child at rest, from afar, and on physical examination, and then the use of a tool that can be measured by scientifically valid scores called rating scales. Only an assessment with a score that is reliable is the one that gives the key to choosing and adapting the prescription [25]. The beliefs of carers, and parents, and misconceptions (for example, "children do not feel as much pain as adults") are a springboard for inadequate pain management [26, 27]. According to the Brazilian Society of Pain Studies (SBED), the main obstacles to pain treatment are inadequate education and training of health professionals, difficulties in pain assessment, lack of knowledge about the pharmacology of opioids and fear of opioids (adverse effects), lack of priority for pain treatment, difficulties in pain reassessment, and proposed treatments [22, 28, 29].

DOI: http://dx.doi.org/10.5772/intechopen.1009125

Awareness-raising and training about children's pain are key to identifying and treating pain by healthcare practitioners. Thus, in our study, the absence of specific signs of pain in the files examined shows the lack of staff knowledge in the assessment and management of pain. The overall knowledge, attitudes, and practices of physicians in our study were below average.

These figures are a logical continuation of the data on knowledge, which was mostly poor due to the lack of training on child pain in front of young professionals with still limited professional experience in the management of infant and small child pain. Indeed, seniority ≥11 years was protective of erroneous attitudes with an odd ratio of 0.03 (0–0.65) and a P value = 0.020. The search for factors influencing inappropriate practices showed that the paediatric grade was protective 0.05 (0–0.82) and a P value of 0.030 of erroneous attitudes and inappropriate practices with an odds ratio of 0 (0–0.47) and a P value of 0.010. Furthermore, in this study, we sought a relationship between inadequate knowledge and wrong attitudes on the one hand between inadequate knowledge and wrong practices on the other hand, and between wrong attitudes and wrong practices on the other. There is a significant relationship between wrong attitudes and inappropriate practices with a P value of 0.04. 58% of our sample had wrong attitudes and inappropriate practices. Insufficient knowledge exposed 1.03 (0.26–4.24) times to improper practices.

6. Limit of study

Throughout this study, we have encountered difficulties with the collaboration of some doctors and the negligence of some carers during the filling of the medical records of the patients.

7. Conclusion

Data from our study show that most healthcare professionals are not trained in the management of children's pain, and the pain assessment tools they mention are not age-appropriate. There is a lack of knowledge about pain in relation to age groups. Specific training on the child's pain is needed in health training.

Acknowledgements

We thank the CME/FCB staff who agreed to participate in this study.

Conflict of interest

The authors declare no conflict of interest.

Author details

Angèle Hermine Pondy Ongotsoyi[1*], Laura Murielle Kuate Makowa[2], Patience Tazanou Ngouanet[3], Louise Loe Renee[4] and Audrey Miyehane[5]

1 Mother and Child Centre, Chantal Biya Foundation, Yaoundé, Cameroon

2 Faculty of Medicine and Biomedical Sciences, University of Yaoundé I, Yaoundé, Cameroon

3 Higher Institute of Medical Technology, Yaoundé, Cameroon

4 Alternative Health, Yaoundé, Cameroon

5 Institute of Medical Technology, Yaoundé, Cameroon

*Address all correspondence to: pondyangeleh@gmail.com

References

[1] American Academy of Paediatrics. Committee on psychosocial aspects of child and family health, task force on pain in infants, children, and adolescents. The assessment and management of acute bread in infants, children, and adolescents. Paediatrics. 2001;**108**:793-797. DOI: 10.1542/peds.108.3.793

[2] Subhashini L, Vatsa M, Lodha R. Knowledge, attitude and practices among health care professionals regarding bread. Indian Journal of Pediatrics. 2009;**76**:913-916. DOI: 10.1007/s12098-009-0154-6

[3] Fitzgerald M. The development of nociceptive circuits. Nature Reviews. Neuroscience. 2005;**6**:507-520. DOI: 10.1038/nrn1701

[4] Srouji R, Ratnapalan S, SchneeweissS.Paininchildren:Assessment and nonpharmacological management. International Journal of Pediatrics. 2010;**2010**:474838. DOI: 10.1155/2010/474838

[5] Beltramini A, Milojevic K, Pateron D. Pain assessment in newborns, infants, and children. Pediatric Annals. 2017;**46**:e387-e395. DOI: 10.3928/19382359-20170921-03

[6] Manworren R, Stinson J. Seminars in paediatric neurology paediatric pain measurement, assessment and evaluation. Seminars in Pediatric Neurology. 2016;**23**:189-200. DOI: 10.1016/j.spen.2016.10.001

[7] José EM, Oudou N. L'Enquête CAP (Connaissances, Attitudes, Pratiques) en Recherche Médicale. 2013;**14**:3

[8] de Gabriel Freitas RM, de Cláudio Castro G Jr, Stela Castro MJ, Heineck I. Degree of knowledge of health care professionals about pain management and use of opioids in paediatrics. Pain Medicine (Malden Mass). 2014;**15**:807-819. DOI: 10.1111/pme.12332

[9] Rappaport L. Recurrent abdominal pain: Theories and pragmatics. Paediatrician. 1989;**16**:78-84

[10] Friedrichsdorf SJ, Postier AC. Recent advances in bread treatment for children with serious illness. Management in Bread. 2019;**9**:583-596. DOI: 10.2217/pmt-2019-0029

[11] Friedrichsdorf SJ, Goubert L. Paediatric pain treatment and prevention for hospitalised children. Schmerz Berl Ger. 2021;**35**:195-210. DOI: 10.1007/s00482-020-00519-0

[12] Sporrer KA, Jackson SM, Agner S, Laver J, Abboud MR. Bread in children and adolescents with sickle cell anaemia: A prospective study utilising self-reporting. The American Journal of Pediatric Hematology/Oncology. 1994;**16**:219-224. DOI: 10.1097/00043426-199408000-00006

[13] Stevens MM, Dalla Pozza L, Cavalletto B, Cooper MG, Kilham HA. Pain and symptom control in paediatric palliative care. Cancer Surveys. 1994;**21**:211-231

[14] Panjganj D, Bevan A. Children's nurses' post-operative pain assessment practices. Nursing Children and Young People. 2016;**28**:29-33. DOI: 10.7748/ncyp.28.5.29.s23

[15] Kim M-H, Park H, Park EC, Park K. Attitude and knowledge of physicians about cancer pain management:

Young doctors of South Korea in their early career. Japanese Journal of Clinical Oncology. 2011;**41**:783-791. DOI: 10.1093/jjco/hyr043

[16] Bourdon O, Brion F. Management of cancer bread in children. Annales Pharmaceutiques En. 2006;**64**:17-22. DOI: 10.1016/s0003-4509(06)75289-0

[17] Fournier-Charrière E, Dommergues JP. Pain in children: Specific aspects. La Revue du Praticien. 1994;**44**:1925-1931

[18] Van Hulle VC. Nurses' knowledge, attitudes, and practices: Regarding children's bread. MCN: American Journal of Maternal Child Nursing. 2005;**30**:177-183. DOI: 10.1097/00005721-200505000-00005

[19] Linhares MBM, Doca FNP, Martinez FE, Carlotti APP, Cassiano RGM, Pfeifer LI, et al. Paediatric pain: Prevalence, assessment, and management in a teaching hospital. Brazilian Journal of Medical and Biological Research. 2012;**45**:1287-1294. DOI: 10.1590/S0100-879X2012007500147

[20] Pancekauskaitė G, Jankauskaitė L. Paediatric pain medicine: Pain differences, recognition and coping acute procedural pain in paediatric emergency room. Medicina (Kaunas, Lithuania). 2018;**54**:E94. DOI: 10.3390/medicina54060094

[21] Boerner KE, Chambers CT, McGrath PJ, LoLordo V, Uher R. The effect of parental modelling on child pain responses: The role of parent and child sex. The Journal of Pain. 2017;**18**:702-715. DOI: 10.1016/j.jpain.2017.01.007

[22] L'évaluation pratique de la douleur chez l'enfant (à propos de 61 malades) – Centre Hospitalier Universitaire Hassan II. n.d. Available from: http://www.chu-fes.ma/levaluation-pratique-de-la-douleur-chez-lenfant-a-propos-de-61-malades/ [Accessed: October 13, 2021]

[23] Stevens BJ, Abbott LK, Yamada J, Harrison D, Stinson J, Taddio A, et al. Epidemiology and management of painful procedures in children in Canadian hospitals. Canadian Medical Association Journal. 2011;**183**:E403-E410. DOI: 10.1503/cmaj.101341

[24] Laures E, LaFond C, Hanrahan K, Pierce N, Min H, McCarthy AM. Pain assessment practices in the paediatric intensive care unit. Journal of Pediatric Nursing. 2019;**48**:55-62. DOI: 10.1016/j.pedn.2019.07.005

[25] Quinn BL, Sheldon LK, Cooley ME. Paediatric pain assessment by drawn faces scales: A review. Pain Management Nursing. 2014;**15**:909-918. DOI: 10.1016/j.pmn.2014.03.004

[26] Schechter NL. The undertreatment of pain in children: An overview. Pediatric Clinics of North America. 1989;**36**:781-794. DOI: 10.1016/S0031-3955(16)36721-9

[27] Walco GA, Cassidy RC, Schechter NL. Bread, hurt, and harm. The ethics of pain control in infants and children. The New England Journal of Medicine. 1994;**331**:541-544. DOI: 10.1056/NEJM199408253310812

[28] Pedroso RA, Celich KLS. Dor: quinto sinal vital, um desafio para o cuidar em enfermagem. Text Contexto - Enferm. 2006;**15**:270-276. DOI: 10.1590/S0104-07072006000200011

[29] Ii Consenso Nacional De Dor Oncológica - PDF Download grátis. n.d. Available from: https://docplayer.com.br/50484685-Ii-consenso-nacional-de-dor-oncologica.html [Accessed: October 13, 2021]

Section 3

Opportunities

Chapter 8

Perspective Chapter: India and Palliative Care – Opportunities and Barriers

Purnima Jain and Constance Dahlin

Abstract

The chapter focuses on the current health model of India and the health infrastructure followed in the country to date. India is a country with linguistic and cultural diversity, and it is replete with distinctive beliefs related to life and death. Being a collectivistic culture with a norm of serving communities, volunteerism has uplifted the country's health needs both during the COVID-19 pandemic and in serving critically ill patients. Pallium India and Accredited Social Health Activist workers have done tremendous work in serving people and communities in the most remote areas of the country. The chapter discusses combining the strength of community-based palliative care and Accredited Social Health Activists to meet the growing need of individuals with serious illnesses and ensuring access to palliative care. The use of advance care planning as a tool to initiate palliative care at the diagnosis of a serious illness rather than at end of life to move palliative care into the community is described. Finally, there is a discussion of the lack of multidisciplinary treatment in palliative care in India, which negatively impacts comprehensive care and quality of life.

Keywords: palliative care, India, pallium India, accredited social health activist, advance care planning, opportunities, barriers

1. Introduction

India is the seventh-largest country by geography and the second-most-populated country in the world [1]. There are 28 states, each with their own governments, and eight union territories governed in part or whole, by the union government of India. Along with being endowed with natural resources, India is known for its economic strategies and politics being the largest democratic country in the world. The country has a rich linguistic and cultural diversity with dialects and rituals changing every 100 km [1].

With such diversity, there are disparate views on life and death. Life and death are phenomena considered as the two sides of the same coin. While there are celebrations and community-level rituals related to birth, there are also rituals associated with death [2]. These rituals are different in different religions that are practiced in India. For birth, it is common to distribute sweets in the neighborhood, donate money or food at religious places, and exchange gifts in the family. For death, there are varying rituals depending on one's religion.

The cultural diversity on death is reflected in the beliefs and rituals of the many religions [2]. The most common religion is Hinduism. Individuals practicing Hinduism prefer to die at home surrounded by loved ones. The end-of-life is associated with detachment from the physical and material world and preparing for death through meditation, prayers. Chanting of *vedic*, Hindu scripture mantras, occur alongside the dying person which is believed to help the family in coping with the loss of the deceased. Statements like "bad deeds conducted in past or present life, God's will, and God recalls back from earth good people" are common narratives that are believed. Additionally, reframing statements like renunciation from material world, and reincarnation to a better life are phrases common among followers of Hinduism that help them cope with bereavement.

Other religions have differing rituals [2]. Individuals practicing Buddhism believe in the concept of reincarnation and detachment from the material world, with a more specific belief in discouraging the use of narcotics at the end-of-life. Individuals who practice Jainism believe that the soul and the physical body are two different entities and that death brings the end of the physical body but not the soul which continues to live. Jainism teaches about attaining *'moksha'* or breaking the cycle of life and death to achieve liberation. Individuals who practice Christianity in India believe in the concept of sin and punishment which is associated with suffering and death. This is accompanied by the belief that soul lives after death. Those practicing Islam, also believe in submission of suffering to the Almighty, but allow the use of opioids to manage severe pain in dying patients. It is essential to understand the beliefs of life and death in India to ensure care for patients with terminal illnesses matches religious perspectives along with influences on the acceptance of palliative care [2].

2. Healthcare delivery

The health care model of India follows a triarchic model (shown graphically in **Figure 1**). The health infrastructure and healthcare system are divided into a three-tier system, namely primary, secondary and tertiary levels [3, 4]. The primary level includes subcenters and primary health centers and is the first point of contact for the community. These centers provide services related to maternal and child health, communicable and non-communicable disease control programs, family planning, health

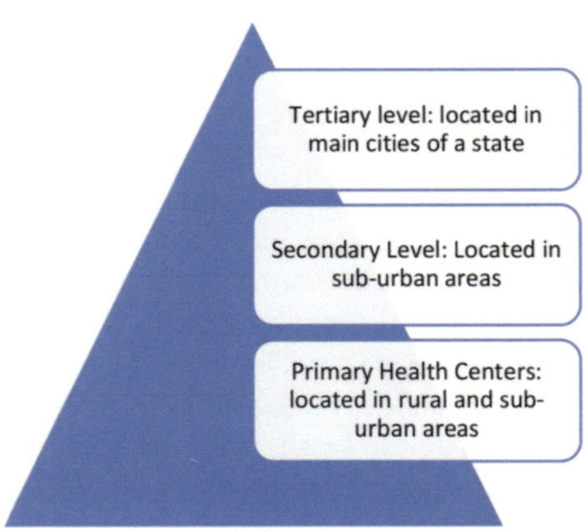

Figure 1.
Healthcare model of India.

education, and basic laboratory services. The secondary level includes community health centers and district hospitals that provide more specialized care. The primary and secondary health centers are located in rural and suburban geographical areas. The tertiary care centers include medical colleges and specialized hospitals, which offer advanced medical services and treatments on 'disease control'.

Despite the efficient three-tiered health system that ensures healthcare needs are met by the population living in the most remote areas, accessibility of the healthcare services is still a challenge. The Indian healthcare sector occupies a modest 2.1% of the Gross Domestic Product (GDP) [5]. This has resulted in a lower density of medical practitioners (1.34 Doctors per 1000 population) [3, 5, 6], a reduced number of hospital beds (5.3 beds per 1000 population) [3, 5, 6], and higher out-of-pocket healthcare expenditures (50.60% of health spending) [2, 5]. India falls short of the World Health Organization (WHO) recommended number of nurses with only 1.96 nurses per 1000 population, which is against the recommended rate of three per 1000 population [7]. Additionally, an increase in the burden of chronic diseases [5, 8], the rise in the aging population [5], and overwhelming health needs (poor maternal-child care, malnutrition, anemia, and increased levels of communicable and non-communicable diseases) [4, 8], desperately necessitate increased scalability of investment in healthcare infrastructure [5].

For Indians, there is a choice of the biomedical model of treatment for pain management and symptom control or traditional healing [9]. Traditional healing, which is more common in rural and tribal communities also uses various ancient healing practices through *Siddha, Unani*, and *Nattu* [10]. These treatment models are embedded in the principles of Ayurveda, and tantric theories and practices. Despite the origin of Unani in Greece, it was embraced by Indians from the twelfth century BC and is now part of the healthcare program of Ayurveda, Yoga, Unani, Naturopathy, and Homeopathy (AYUSH) [9–11]. The healthcare program of AYUSH was implemented under the purview of the National Rural Health Mission of the Ministry of Health to provide services related to alternative medicine [11]. As previously stated, India falls short of healthcare professionals in comparison to its growing need to serve the population [3, 5, 6]. Thus, the Ministry of health streamlined the AYUSH to meet the challenge of the shortage of healthcare professionals and for strengthening the healthcare services [11].

Even with the promotion of AYUSH by the government as a holistic approach to treatment, physicians and nurses do not integrate it as adjunct therapy to modern medicines for either communicable diseases or non-communicable diseases [9]. However, yoga and breathing exercises like *Pranayama* have been promoted by both the medical society and the government alike for management of hypertension and diabetes [9–11]. Alternatively, separate from AYUSH, traditional healers are recognized by tribal communities across India. These healers deliver ritualistic and non-ritualistic practices from knowledge of local herbs that have been passed down from generations [12].

The pervasiveness of traditional healing is increasing whether among urban, metropolitan cities to remote, rural areas [12]. Mapping of these traditional healers is a task in itself. The last credible census data is from 1992, and it reveals that more than half a million healers, which is assumed to have increased over the years [10]. However, independent studies conducted in the states of Rajasthan, Madhya Pradesh, Chhattisgarh, and Jharkhand have recorded high numbers of traditional healers. Traditional healing is a hope for patients and families when modern medicine fails to provide symptom relief [9–11]. The government of India along with the WHO established 'Global Centre for Traditional Medicine' in Jamnagar, India in 2022 with an investment of $250 million U.S. dollars [12]. The aim of this program is research on traditional healing and maximizing its effectiveness through modern science and technology.

Despite the government's endless efforts and initiatives to make healthcare services available to even the most remote areas of the country, there is an absence of an integrated care and interdisciplinary service delivery model affecting the quality of care [4]. According to the WHO 2022, India ranks high in premature deaths from non-communicable diseases [3, 13–16]. This accounts for 60% of all deaths in India [13, 17]. Moreover, it has been suggested that the unwarranted fragmentation of healthcare with the three-tier system without an integrated care model had led to negative outcomes within an already overburdened tertiary healthcare organization [18]. These include an increase in medical errors and misdiagnoses, along with provider burnout due to an increase in self-referral to tertiary care when many of the services could be provided at the primary level [3, 4, 18].

There is further pressure due to the current health model of India on tertiary care due to its emphasis on 'saving lives' [18] and health infrastructure putting efforts toward increasing longevity with the absence of equal efforts toward caring for terminal illness [3, 4, 15]. This has resulted in increased personal or family out-of-pocket expenditures which creates financial instability [15]. India ranks low, 67 out of 80 countries, in the *Quality of Death Index,* reflecting the country's struggle to provide accessible and high-quality palliative care [19]. Patients who are dying experience prolonged advanced illnesses with multiple hospitalizations and long periods of home bed confinement [3, 13, 14, 16, 20]. The multidisciplinary approach involving physicians, nurses, social workers, mental health practitioners, and traditional healers has yet to be implemented [16]. This is because of the focus on the biomedical model of end-of-life care, which restricts services to just pain management and symptom control.

Community-based palliative care, which provides services through multidisciplinary treatment, and the involvement of an Accredited Social Health Activist (ASHA) are two untapped potentials that can not only reduce the burden on tertiary care but can also reduce financial burdens and facilitate the emotional well-being of patients and their families who are grappling with critical illnesses.

3. Health model

The health model of India, currently, has a huge investment in 'saving lives', specifically focusing on curative treatment [9]. For example, there is a major focus on tuberculosis (TB) due to its high incidence, resulting in the government of India (GOI) mission to eradicate it by 2030 [6]. TB treatment is available for free at all government and registered private and Non-Governmental Organization (NGO) health facilities. Similarly, HIV treatment has been kept within the economic reach of daily wage workers [6, 21, 22]. Additionally, several international medical humanitarian organizations like Doctors without Borders and the Gates Foundation have been working rigorously in adding India's efforts toward eradicating communicable and vector-borne diseases [23].

The country's health infrastructure is continuously witnessing a health revolution, with low-cost medical devices, innovative healthcare delivery models, and healthcare services at comparatively low costs [5]. This attracts international health tourism for patients seeking quality treatment at affordable prices. Private healthcare providers are investing significantly in developing modern hospitals, clinics, and diagnostic centers equipped with advanced medical technology. To circumscribe the problem of geographical distance between rural and urban areas, the current healthcare system counterbalances the hindrance to healthcare access by using a telehealth infrastructure and access to smartphone devices. With the availability of affordable telehealth programs, including access to 5G data for as low as $4.12 per month, India ranks second in the world for smartphone use. The health infrastructure has capitalized on easy and affordable telehealth services to revolutionize healthcare access in the most remote areas, as even the most remote areas have access to WhatsApp [24]. This has enabled the implementation of digital innovations such as electronic medical records, telemedicine, health apps, and remote monitoring systems to improve patient care. Increased health insurance coverage has enabled access to private healthcare services, with insurance companies collaborating with private hospitals and clinics [5].

The rising health needs of the population are promoting preventative health care in India. This includes fitness, wellness, nutrition, vitamins and mineral supplements, early diagnostics, and health tracking. The preventative healthcare sector is expected to reach $197 billion in 2025 with the compound annual growth rate (CAGR) of 22% [5] as compared to 12.2% for cancer between the years 2023 and 2028 [6], 4% for mycobacterium tuberculosis through 2033 [25], 5.08% for HIV/AIDS treatment for Lopinavir and Ritonavir and 6.54% between 2024 and 2032 [21, 22]. All this data demonstrates that India has parallel investments initiated in the preventative healthcare sector.

The rising incidences of chronic and non-communicable diseases like diabetes, thyroid conditions, hypertension, and heart disease, are facilitating the adoption of preventative healthcare [5]. Efforts to eradicate polio, tuberculosis, new HIV infection, and other vector-borne diseases are being achieved through collaboration with international NGOs. Healthcare start-ups are proliferating with global and local investments of over US $150 million. These start-ups are working in the fields of nutrition, wellness, and genomics to name a few areas. The result is increased vaccination drives, broader immunization programs, TB treatment, cancer treatment, and malnutrition treatment, which are all provided free of cost/minimal expenditure through government-aided hospitals, irrespective of socio-economic status [3, 5]. Therefore, for a country with a huge population, health infrastructure is more inclined toward prevention than cure to increase longevity.

With curative and preventative measures receiving increased attention from the government and private sector healthcare organizations, palliative care has yet to receive equal focused attention. Government coverage of hospice and palliative care is still in its rudimentary stage as the focus of healthcare programs is more on prevention and cure to keep people healthier with improved rates of longevity [8]. This again reflects the idea that the notion of health is pushing away death, hence, there is more need to focus on death and dying by embracing the idea of hospice and palliative care. Since its inception in 1986 as 'Shanti Avedna Sadan' in Mumbai [2], palliative care has been under the realm of NGOs and individual efforts with advocacy by motivated physicians, lawyers, nurses, and community health workers [26]. The availability of palliative care is still skewed in India with many activities in south India have been initiated by Pallium India in 2003 under the leadership of Dr. M.R. Rajagopal [27].

Before discussing barriers and opportunities, it is important to understand the notion of death and how it is perceived in the current healthcare infrastructure. As previously stated, India's healthcare structure is viewed through the lenses of longevity and prolonging lifespan. The result is an increase in the average life expectancy from age 32 in 1947 post-independence from colonialism to approximately age 67 in 2024 in a free and independent India [24]. Early diagnosis and quick treatment are the precursors for increasing the lifespan [5, 24]. However, there is still a significant proportion of the population inflicted with terminal illness, with the rate increasing annually. It is estimated that each year in India, there are 1 million diagnoses of cancer, with over 80% occurring at stages III and IV [2, 16, 17]. It is estimated that the annual total number of patients who need palliative care is likely to be 6 million people [17]. These estimates include the paucity of prompt availability of medical treatment or diagnosis [5], lack of health literacy within the public [8], and/or treatment failure as delivered by physicians [19].

A multidisciplinary treatment approach should be more streamlined similar to AYUSH through government initiatives. This requires medical education and awareness initiating research into developing multidisciplinary treatment as a standard of practice [17, 19]. Thus, care should be comprehensive, not just nursing care, pain management, and symptom control [27], but include social work and mental health to address the social welfare and emotional well-being of patients and families. Bereavement counseling also needs to be included as a part of the standard care model for palliative care [23].

4. Palliative care

India has various factors that necessitate the implementation of palliative care across the country [13]. These factors include rising rates of patients with serious illnesses, an increase in the aging population, an increase in financial instability from health care expenditure, and a lack of palliative care education and training programs [14]. The notion of comfort or palliative care is poorly understood. It is either viewed as a luxury or if available, mostly accepted or present in large urban settings with a solid health infrastructure. The result is a skewed availability of palliative care services across the country. Within metropolitan cities like Delhi, Mumbai, and Calcutta, palliative care services are restricted to pain management and nursing care with little scope for holistic care for mental health, bereavement counseling, or spiritual care [20, 25, 28]. Those living in urban and high socio-economic status opt for nursing care in home-based palliative care. The nurse's role is that of being relegated to personal care and assisting with activities of daily living. However, access to palliative care services in rural areas is restricted [20, 25, 27]. For individuals living in rural areas, which is three quarters of the population [8], the onus of care lies with family members. Those family members who are responsible are the nonearning members of the family; mostly women and young children because men are daily wage workers.

According to the *Global Atlas of Palliative Care*, palliative care and end-of-life care needs in the south-east Asian region (SEAR) is estimated to be around 175–275/100,000 population [14, 16]. As already mentioned earlier, the quality of death in India is among the lowest ranks. Additional data shows that the capacity to deliver palliative and end-of-life care scored as low as 0.6/100 [14, 17]. This means that only 0.4% of the population in India has access to palliative and end-of-life care [2, 13, 21, 22]. According to the *Quality of Death Index Report*, poor quality of end-of-life care delivery in India has been kept at the periphery of the current health model [20]. Along with the lack of training in palliative care for health professionals, shortage of palliative care specialists or subject matter experts, and poor public awareness

Barriers to Palliative Care in India	Lack of training in palliative care of health professionals
	Shortage of palliative care specialists or subject matter experts
	Poor public awareness on palliative and end-of-life care

Table 1.
Palliative care barriers in India.

of palliative and end-of-life care, are barriers to the implementation of national level palliative care [8, 20]. Thus, to meet the growing population's needs, it is essential to promulgate the belief that palliative care is not a luxury. It is a fundamental right where compassion and quality of care for patients with serious illness take center stage (**Table 1**) [19].

Access to palliative care services in rural areas is scare, hindered by the workforce at the grassroots level [8, 29]. Traveling from remote areas to palliative care services is difficult because there is inadequate transportation. Along with inadequate infrastructure and scarcity of skilled healthcare workers, lack of awareness or knowledge of palliative care further impedes acceptance and implications of palliative care [8, 13, 20]. Families in rural areas invest emotionally and financially in treatment with the goal of cure. They may often mortgage their physical resources whether it is their house, agricultural land, or lending money from friends, or local moneylenders or *sahukars* who charge high rates of interest to continue treatment. Consequently, they view palliative care as when physicians have given up on the patient. Families of patients diagnosed with HIV/AIDS face the double burden of high financial burdens and subsequent stigma and discrimination [22, 23]. Thus, receiving an incurable, serious illness, diagnosis from a health team disheartens the family. Health professionals often hear statements such as, "*Please do everything to save our loved one, please continue with the treatment, if God wants to save the patient, He will; we have prayed a lot to Almighty, we know He will not fail us; we have done good deeds, God will not punish us like this; can you make the patient the way he was before being sick*". It is not a matter of rectifying the belief system of the population toward palliative care or death and dying but it is about providing the required support.

5. Current palliative care infrastructure

Pallium India is one such organization based on the concept of community-based palliative care. Founded in 2003 by Dr. M.R. Rajagopal [2], the organization has been working tirelessly with national and international organizations to provide pain management to patients. Additionally, the organization is acclaimed internationally for the inclusion of community healthcare workers who provide counseling, health management, and rehabilitation services for patients, and supportive care to patients' families [30]. Initially started in Kerala, located in south India, Pallium India has a 20-year history of activities in Jharkhand, Tripura, Uttar Pradesh, Manipur, Mizoram, Bihar, Orissa, Gujarat, Meghalaya, Tamil Nadu, and Lakshadweep. Additionally, to meet much-needed capacity building within palliative and end-of-life care, Pallium India has developed three learning centers in three different Indian cities [4]: Trivandrum, Jaipur, and Ahmedabad. Education and training focus on communication, conflict resolution, end-of-life care, pediatric care, clinical issues related to anorexia, cachexia, fatigue, legal issues, prognostication, and dealing with difficult patients [30].

Another area of focus for Pallium India has been its ongoing public awareness campaign. This includes get-togethers for patients, arts and crafts exhibitions, food festivals, and cultural events to spread the message of palliative care [2, 27]. The state of Kerala observes 15th January annually as a day for "Compassionate Communities-together for palliative care" [27, 30]. Within the past 20 years, Pallium India has successfully instilled local awareness of palliative care resulting in a high number of Pallium India community volunteers who provide holistic care to patients with home-based palliative care through its program named 'Neighborhood Network in Palliative Care' [2]. It has also instilled the message to the health community and the general public that palliative care is a service model at any stage of the illness, alongside curative treatment, not just treatment for dying patients. Care includes pain and symptom relief and emotional support. Pallium India's home-based palliative care serves as a role model for prospective palliative care services globally.

Pallium India, under the leadership of Dr. Rajagopal, also participates in advocacy and research. For example, it is estimated that annually around 7 million patients with advanced cancer, and non-cancer medical conditions like HIV/AIDS, and other incurable, progressive diseases, experience moderate to severe pain at any given time [17, 27]. Unfortunately, only 4% of these patients have access to pain medications due to stringent laws related to the procurement of licenses by medical hospitals and medical professionals for access to morphine for pain relief [13, 14, 17, 27]. This has limited access to morphine, even if palliative care services are provided in a hospital. Therefore, in 2013, Pallium India initiated its advocacy program named 'Morphine Manifesto' [17]. This advocacy program asserts toward improving safe access toward release of oral morphine. Their efforts have been on working with the Central and State Governments to remove the regulatory barriers to opioid access.

Pallium India views advocacy as essential to bring much-needed change and sensitivity for medical and non-medical needs for patients with life-limiting medical conditions [27]. This gained the attention of the international palliative care community, resulting in 63 international communities signing up to collaborate on the 'Morphine Manifesto' [17]. Without structured government guidelines on palliative and end-of-life care, the organization continuously collaborates with national and international experts on palliative care to establish national standards, that is, minimum standards for palliative care programs for ensuring quality palliative care [27].

Due to its achievements, Pallium India has received nationally and internationally recognition. With its credibility, it could play an instrumental role in the movement toward multidisciplinary treatment. This would involve increasing the development of palliative care by the inclusion of subject matter experts on mental health and traditional healing. Even though the government has advocated for mental health, removing the stigma associated with mental health issues [29]. However, counseling and psychological first aid are still associated with and restricted to the Psychiatry Department at any government or private hospitals and lack connection to critical care departments.

Doctors without Borders medical program on Advanced HIV at Patna, Bihar, is an outlier to multidisciplinary care [23]. The organization has a 30-bed hospital dedicated to the treatment of advanced HIV and has a strong component of palliative care through multidisciplinary treatment. This program includes health promotion and mental health teams who work tirelessly, providing comfort care to patients dying from HIV while simultaneously removing the stigma and discrimination associated with HIV. Thus, the health team should include not just physicians and nurses but also mental health counselors, health promotion/social workers, anthropologists, and pharmacists.

Team meetings are held on a weekly basis and include case discussions and identifying patients and families who would benefit from care. Care comprises of conjoint sessions co-facilitated by the teams, using the SPIKES model to frame breaking difficult news. Patients and families have reported that the support from care provided by Doctors without Borders helped them recognize that one deserves respect and dignity irrespective of the treatment outcome. This program is a critically acclaimed program, setting the milestone for further research in palliative care.

India is a country with a collectivist culture with emotions taking a primary place in decision-making and guiding one's behavior. Serving the community is a humanitarian principle across different religions [2]. This principle has given rise to palliative care and ASHA workers in India [28]. ASHA workers are mainly women from middle to low socio-economic status with high school graduation degrees. Their main objective is to serve the community and receive some compensation (although no basic monthly salary) in exchange for the services undertaken by them. There are currently over 1 million of these workers who are connecting the rural population to the primary health centers [15, 28]. With such strong emphasis and values placed on the importance of serving the community, integration of palliative care in primary health centers through the use of ASHA workers could be efficient and effective.

Their work in caring for individuals with serious illnesses was demonstrated during the COVID-19 pandemic. ASHA workers played a critical role in amplifying the country's efforts toward COVID-19 vaccination by ensuring required prevention reaches to the most remote areas of the country. ASHA workers provided psychological support and education to the rural and suburban population with infection prevention control measures (IPC) against the spread of the virus, which was a serious and life-threatening illness. Their role during the COVID-19 pandemic was pertinent and instrumental in controlling the spread of virus in the rural areas. In 2022, WHO recognized the ASHAs in the 75th World Health Assembly for their relentless efforts to serve the community during the pandemic [31].

Therefore, because of the intrinsic motivation within the ASHA workers to serve the community, their access to the rural population, and their experience with serious and life-threatening illnesses, they would benefit from specialized palliative care education and training through an acclaimed organizations like Pallium India. With such education and training ASHA workers could provide palliative care services, including pain management through analgesics, emotional support, and spiritual care in the rural communities they are part of.

Bereavement counseling, which is still a missing piece in the majority of palliative care programs, could be available if adequate training was provided to the ASHA workers. One research study reported that in order for community-based palliative care to be integrated into society, the inclusion of grassroots workers like ASHAs would ensure that patients with end-of-life diseases and their families would not be abandoned to cope without any support [15].

6. Advance care planning

Another area that would further ensure that palliative care is provided at the early onset of the disease is through advance care planning (ACP). ACP as part of palliative care involves patient preferences for goals of care, pain and symptom management, declining or discontinuing treatment, cultural and spiritual support, and preferred place of death. Within the context of India, the Mental Health Care Act (2017, 2018) formalized the use of ACP codified as Advance Directive (AD), which is a document containing decisions made by a patient, or proxy toward the treatment with the primary health care provider [26, 29]. ACP is an evolving process and empowers patients by documenting their wishes based on expectations toward treatment [26]. Patients diagnosed with life-limiting medical conditions are encouraged to choose a substitute decision-maker and document their health and care preferences in an advance care directive [29]. Moreover, ACP eases the financial burden on the patient and family by pulling back active treatment gradually when it is no longer medically beneficial to the patient.

However, ACP has been underutilized. This could be attributed to factors that include government-initiated legislation that delays the ease of implementation of ACP, poor prognostication (e.g., fear of committing errors at detecting poor prognosis), fear of litigation by the patient's families, or poor patient-physician ratio which hampers communication between patient and families [26].

A few programs with a multidisciplinary model of treatment such as the HIV/AIDS program of Doctors without Borders, use ACP as a document, where conversations during the conjoint sessions co-facilitated by the team with patient/family are recorded [23]. Treatment decisions such as do-not-resuscitate (DNR), informed consent for invasive procedures like lumbar puncture, ICU care, conversations focusing on comfort care rather than curative treatment, preferred place of death (whether hospital or home) are discussed and recorded through ACP document. It should be noted that the use of nasogastric tubes has cultural concerns and is not easily accepted in Indian communities, hence consent is required.

ACP for life-limiting medical conditions, is regarded as a tool to ensure a person-centered approach with its possible result in reducing the incidences of leaving against medical advice (LAMA) [32]. Physicians and intensivists believe that aligning the patient's values with the available treatment options would ensure their satisfaction and agreement with the medical team [26, 32]. Even though the concept of discontinuing and withholding of care are influenced by local cultural traditions and norms, ACP performed effectively would ensure that the patients and their families trust treatment, which could lead to improved adherence [26]. It has been demonstrated that education and training of physicians on ACP is important as results in improved communication between them and the patients leading to more acceptance and awareness of ACP.

7. Conclusion

India is a diverse country rich in culture and languages which change every 100 kilometers. Being the most populous country in the world with a population of over a billion people, there are myriad ideologies on life and death. Being a collectivistic culture, it places value on emotions rather than logic when engaging in important decisions. This value has influenced the country's acceptance of palliative care. Young health professionals whose focus is more on 'saving lives' along with the community in general often regard palliative care as a luxury or a process that hastens death. The health infrastructure of the country places huge investments on prevention, and then on curative treatment. Increasing longevity is one of the indicators of economic growth. Despite its focus on 'saving lives' model of care, local movements bringing awareness toward palliative care have received recognition and collaboration from not only national leaders but also from international organizations as well.

DOI: http://dx.doi.org/10.5772/intechopen.1009282

There is a movement to improve care for individuals with serious illness at end of life. The Indian government is collaborating with both Indian and international NGOs. Pallium India has been igniting efforts in bringing palliative care to the forefront. ASHA workers are promising front-line workers who, when provided with the required training and capacity building on palliative care, would increase the availability and access for patients in remote areas of the country. International NGOs like Doctors without Borders are working tirelessly to bringing palliative care to patients who are stigmatized and discriminated due to their illness. Physicians, lawyers, and social workers are recognizing the importance of ACP as a valid tool to ensure more person-centered care to patients dealing with progressive diseases. The result is patient's right and dignity even at the end-of-life is safeguarded by honoring their choices and decisions. In summary, there are many inroads to palliative care in India, from primary level care to tertiary care, that will increase access to care of the needs of growing and culturally diverse population in the community.

Author details

Purnima Jain[1*] and Constance Dahlin[1,2,3*]

1 University of Maryland Baltimore, School of Graduate Studies Graduate Studies in Palliative Care, Baltimore, MD, USA

2 Center to Advance Palliative Care, New York, NY, United States

3 MGB Salem Hospital, Salem, MA, United States

*Address all correspondence to: purnima.jain@umaryland.edu and aprneducation@gmail.com

References

[1] Naraya H. India, a Land of Many Tongues. The Hindu. 21 Apr 2021. Available from: https://www.thehindu.com/thread/arts-culture-society/india-a-land-of-many-tongues/article19445187.ece [Accessed: April 6, 2025]

[2] Mir WA, Misra S, Sanghavi D. Life before death in India: A narrative review. Indian Journal of Palliative Care. 2023;**29**(2):207

[3] Kumar A. The transformation of the Indian healthcare system. Cureus. 16 May 2023;**15**(5)

[4] Mirza M, Verma M, Aggarwal A, Satpathy S, Sahoo SS, Kakkar R. Indian model of integrated healthcare (IMIH): A conceptual framework for a coordinated referral system in resource-constrained settings. BMC Health Services Research. 2024;**24**(1):42

[5] Jain D. The Rise of Preventive Healthcare in India. The Times of India; 3 Jan 2023. Available from: https://timesofindia.indiatimes.com/blogs/voices/the-rise-of-preventive-healthcare-in-india/ [Accessed: April 6, 2025]

[6] Sinha P, Carwile M, Bhargava A, Cintron C, Acuna-Villaorduna C, Lakshminarayan S, et al. How much do Indians pay for tuberculosis treatment? A cost analysis. Public Health Action. 2020;**10**(3):110-117

[7] Press Times India. Shortage of Nurses in India, their Emigration for Jobs Abroad Cause of Worry: Experts. 22 May 2024. Available from: https://www.ptinews.com/story/national/shortage-of-nurses-in-india-their-emigration-for-jobs-abroad-cause-of-worry-experts/1523478 [Accessed: April 6, 2025]

[8] Atreya S, Datta S, Salins N. Public health perspective of primary palliative care: A review through the lenses of general practitioners. Indian Journal of Palliative Care. 2022;**28**(3):229

[9] Ojha A, Ojha U, Ojha H, Chandrashekar A, Mohammed R, Trivedi R, et al. Role of AYUSH therapies in modern medicine: A qualitative study to explore the awareness and attitudes of doctors towards the utilization of alternate system of medicine for diabetes mellitus. International Journal of General Medicine. 13 Jan 2020:1-8

[10] Fenzel B. Health in India - Healing with Amulets and Antibiotics. Max-Planck-Research; Sep 2011. Available from: https://www.mpg.de/4435613/health-system-india [Accessed: April 5, 2025]

[11] Shrivastava SR, Shrivastava PS, Ramasamy J. Mainstreaming of Ayurveda, yoga, naturopathy, Unani, siddha, and homeopathy with the health care delivery system in India. Journal of Traditional and Complementary Medicine. 2015;**5**(2):116-118

[12] World Health Organization. WHO Establishes the Global Centre for Traditional Medicine in India. 25 Mar 2022. Available from: https://www.who.int/news/item/25-03-2022-who-establishes-the-global-centre-for-traditional-medicine-in-india [Accessed: April 6, 2025]

[13] Gaikwad A, Acharya S. The future of palliative treatment in India: A review. Cureus. 23 Sep 2022;**14**(9)

[14] Khosla D, Patel FD, Sharma SC. Palliative care in India: Current progress and future needs. Indian Journal of Palliative Care. 2012;**18**(3):149

[15] Prajitha KC, Subbaraman MR, Siddharth Raman SR, Sharahudeen A, Chandran D, Sawyer J, et al. Need of community-based palliative care in rural India and factors that influence its sustainability: A comprehensive exploration using qualitative methodology in rural Puducherry, India. Palliative Care and Social Practice. 2023;**17**:26323524231196315

[16] Salins N, Johnson J, Macaden S. Feasibility and acceptability of implementing the integrated care plan for the dying in the Indian setting: Survey of perspectives of Indian palliative care providers. Indian Journal of Palliative Care. 2017;**23**(1):3

[17] Sharma DC. Morphine manifesto seeks to boost access to oral morphine. The Lancet Oncology. 1 Jan 2024;**25**(1):e5

[18] Myatra SN, Salins N, Iyer S, Macaden SC, Divatia JV, Muckaden M, et al. End-of-life care policy: An integrated care plan for the dying: A joint position statement of the Indian Society of Critical Care Medicine (ISCCM) and the Indian Association of Palliative Care (IAPC). Indian Journal of Critical Care Medicine: Peer-Reviewed, Official Publication of Indian Society of Critical Care Medicine. 2014;**18**(9):615

[19] Vijayender PS. Palliative Care: Where India Stands in the 'Business of Compassion'. ISB Max Institute of Healthcare Management. AMPH Student Blogs. 15 Apr 2024. Available from: https://blogs.isb.edu/healthcare/2024/04/15/palliative-care-where-india-stands-in-the-business-of-compassion/#:~:text=Palliative%20care%20is%20slowly%20gaining,end%2Dof%2Dlife%20journey [Accessed: April 6, 2025]

[20] Chandra A, Debnath A, Nongkynrih B. Palliative care need in India: A systematic review and meta-analysis. Indian Journal of Palliative Care. 2023;**29**(4):375

[21] Future Market Insights. HIV Antivirals Market Outlook (2022 to 2032). Available from: https://www.futuremarketinsights.com/reports/hiv-antivirals-market [Accessed: April 6, 2025]

[22] Kumarasamy N, Venkatesh KK, Mayer KH, Freedberg K. Financial burden of health services for people with HIV/AIDS in India. Indian Journal of Medical Research. 2007;**126**(6):509-517

[23] Medicine San Frontieres. Providing Comprehensive Care to People Living with Advanced-HIV in Bihar. Available from: https://msfsouthasia.org/project/providing-comprehensive-care-to-people-living-with-advanced-hiv-in-bihar/ [Accessed: April 6, 2025]

[24] Macrotrends. India Life Expectancy 1950-2024. Available from: https://www.macrotrends.net/global-metrics/countries/IND/india/life-expectancy [Accessed: April 6, 2025]

[25] MarkNtel. Market Insights and Analysis: India Cancer Treatment Drugs Market (2023-230). Available from: https://www.marknteladvisors.com/research-library/india-cancer-treatment-market.html [Accessed: April 6, 2025]

[26] Indian Association of Palliative Care. Advance Medical Directives and Withdrawal of Life Support Treatment. Webinar; 2023. Available from: https://www.palliativecare.in/webinar-on-advance-medical-directives-and-withdrawal-of-life-support-treatment-on-21st-march-2023/ [Accessed: April 6, 2025]

[27] Rajagopal MR, Joad AK, Muckaden M, George R, Gupta H,

Leng ME, et al. Creation of minimum standard tool for palliative care in India and self-evaluation of palliative care programs using it. Indian Journal of Palliative Care. 2014;**20**(3):201

[28] Pai RR, Nayak MG, Serrao AJ, Salins N. Integrating palliative care into primary health care: Indian perspectives. Progress in Palliative Care. 2023;**31**(5):282-286

[29] Mani RK, Simha S, Gursahani R. Simplified legal procedure for end-of-life decisions in India: A new dawn in the care of the dying? Indian Journal of Critical Care Medicine: Peer-reviewed, Official Publication of Indian Society of Critical Care Medicine. 2023;**27**(5):374

[30] Refresher Course on Palliative Care in Jaipur, India. Available from: https://aphn.org/refresher-course-on-palliative-care-in-jaipur-india/

[31] National Health System. ASHAs - Awarded WHO Director- General's Global Health Leaders Award- 2022 at the 75th World Health Assembly. Available from: https://nhsrcindia.org/ashas-awarded-who-director-generals-global-health-leaders-award-2022-75th-world-health-assembly [Accessed: April 6, 2025]

[32] Paul G, Gautam PL, Mahajan RK, Gautam N, Ragavaiah S. Patients leaving against medical advice-a national survey. Indian Journal of Critical Care Medicine: Peer-Reviewed, Official Publication of Indian Society of Critical Care Medicine. 2019;**23**(3):143

Chapter 9

Care from Strangers: The Development of EoLC Volunteers in Hong Kong

Zhuyun Lin, Gloria Ka-Ming Chun, Felix Fung-Yu Mak, Victoria Ka-Ying Hui and Vivian W.Q. Lou

Abstract

The role of EoLC volunteers is becoming increasingly important globally but is often overlooked in compassionate community building. This chapter explores strategies for developing EoLC volunteers in Hong Kong and enhancing their impact within a compassionate community framework. Our findings show that project-based initiatives and systematic training equip volunteers with essential skills to provide EoLC and organize supportive community activities. Acting as vital connectors between the community and healthcare system, they design and implement care tailored to the needs of patients and families. In this role, volunteers offer practical, psychosocial, spiritual, and physical support to patients and families, improving their quality of life in the final stages and ensuring they do not face these challenges alone. Volunteers gain coping strategies, personal growth, and a deeper sense of purpose. EoLC volunteering also creates strong support networks that reduce the stigma around death and dying, fostering a more informed and compassionate community.

Keywords: compassionate communities, end-of-life care, development strategies, volunteer, Hong Kong

1. Introduction

The growing elderly population globally has focused increasing attention on the importance of maintaining quality of life during the final stages of their lives [1, 2]. Typically, people receiving end-of-life care (EoLC) have a life expectancy of less than 12 months [3]. The primary goal of EoLC is to enhance a patient's quality of life (QoL) in physical, psychosocial, and spiritual aspects, while honoring their healthcare treatment choices [4]. However, research has shown that there is a global deficit of healthcare professionals skilled in EoLC [2, 5, 6]. Moreover, the families, who often act as primary caregivers for the dying person, may not receive sufficient support to undertake EoLC tasks [7]. Providing EoLC to patients and their families thus requires holistic and coordinated efforts from both medical and non-medical teams. While professional care is an essential component, support from the community can enhance the quality of EoLC and help patients achieve a "good death" [8, 9].

Incorporating volunteers into EoLC, especially within community contexts, has been globally recognized as an important strategy to address the deficit created by the increasing demand for services and the decreasing availability of healthcare professionals [10, 11]. Volunteers are generally perceived as providing voluntary assistance in an organized way, to individuals to whom volunteers have no personal obligations [12]. In response to the shortage of manpower in EoLC, volunteers have emerged as key players, providing essential support to professional healthcare services [13]. Volunteers typically function in three ways [14]: as a bridge of connection between patients, families, and healthcare providers; as associates of the healthcare support teams; and as mobile healers. In recognition of the role of volunteers in this area, governments and leading palliative care and hospice associations in countries globally have promoted the volunteering movement and established standards for EoLC volunteer services [15, 16].

1.1 Engaging in compassionate community construction globally

Researches to date show that involving volunteers in EoLC not only helps patients and their families but also contributes to building compassionate communities. Compassionate communities refer to networks of community support that are empowered to improve the well-being of those individuals facing the challenges of serious illness, death, dying, and loss while viewing these experiences as inherent aspects of everyday life [13]. Since its first conceptualization by Allan Kellehear [17], the compassionate community as a public health approach is now gaining momentum all over the world [18–25]. Some examples are described in **Table 1**, demonstrating the many ways in which this approach has been operationalized through volunteers. Several interventions have involved the mobilization of community-based resources and network of care by trained volunteers to support palliative patients and their families [15, 26, 27], filling the gaps in the formal healthcare system where connections between medical and social care are lacking or have been disrupted [14, 33].

The significant role that volunteers play within compassionate communities, particularly in the specialized field of palliative care services, has been universally acknowledged. However, there remains a lack of clarity regarding how volunteers can best contribute to, and lead in, the provision of EoLC under the framework of compassionate community. Addressing this gap, our recent study in Hong Kong proposes a novel approach: *volunteer collaborative leadership* [14]. This approach not only emphasizes volunteers as integral collaborators within a multidisciplinary care team but also positions them as leaders in fostering community connections. Our study aims to demonstrate how this model of improving the quality of EoLC for patients and their families ultimately contributes to building a compassionate Hong Kong. In the following sections, we detail our methods for integrating volunteers into professional care teams and promoting their leadership roles within compassionate communities.

1.2 EoLC volunteers in Hong Kong historically

In Hong Kong, volunteer contributions to EoLC began in the 1950s with missionaries providing spiritual care. From the 1960s to the mid-1980s, healthcare professionals, such as doctors and nurses, volunteered their time to offer mostly spiritual and informal services. Significant progress occurred from the mid-1980s to mid-2000s with the establishment of non-profit organizations like the Society for the Promotion

Countries	India	Australia	UK	Canada
Volunteer-engaged intervention	The Neighborhood Network in Palliative Care [25, 26]	The Compassionate Communities Connectors program [20, 22, 27]	End-of-Life Social Action study [15, 28]	Navigation: Connecting, Assessing, Resourcing, and Engaging [9, 29–31]
Initiator	The Pain and Palliative Care Society	The South West Compassionate Communities Network in Western Australia	The UK Cabinet Office	A 2-year trial of nurse navigation to provide early palliative care [32]
Time period	Since 1993	2020–2022	2015–2016	2015–2016
Number of trained volunteers	Over 10,000 by 2010	20 connectors (2020–2022)	Information not available	Seven (2015–2016); 87 (2018–2021)
Volunteer training	Improve skills in caring for the chronically ill	2-day training; focus on communication, knowledge about services in the community, the importance of network building and network enhancement in supporting patients	Training on boundaries, communication skills and organizational policies according to the requirements of the participating organization	3-day workshop; a navigation curriculum covering six competencies
Volunteer role	Provide social, spiritual, practical (including nursing tasks), and emotional support for patients and family; involve in administration and fund raising; organize awareness programmes in the community	Identify the extra support that patients might need from patients' existing families, friends, neighbors, or local community members who are willing and able to help deliver the support	Offer face-to-face, one-to-one, home-based, non-clinical support (e.g., befriending, practical support, and signposting)	Conduct in-home visits with the patients every three to four weeks over the course of a year to help connect them to the community resources and information they needed
Service target	People with chronic and incurable diseases needing palliative and long-term care at home in rural areas (over 2500 patient beneficiaries per week by 2010); their family	Patients with advanced life-limiting illnesses and who are likely to die within the next 12 months (43 patient beneficiaries by 2022); their family carers	Patients who were expected to die within a year (92 patient beneficiaries by 2016); their family member or informal carer	Older adults with serious illnesses residing in rural communities (23 patient beneficiaries between 2015 and 2016; 50 patient beneficiaries between 2018 and 2021); their family caregivers
Liaison with other stakeholders	Medical staff, local and national government, schools and universities, religious groups, and non-governmental organizations	Caring helpers in the community (e.g., family members, friends, neighbors, or other local citizens), palliative care providers	Participating sites run by national organization, hospices, charity	Nurse navigator who provides an oversight and mentoring role, healthcare providers, other service providers (e.g., legal, home support, transportation, advance care planning, and senior resources)

Table 1.
Examples of volunteer-engaged interventions in supporting a compassionate community approach to palliative care.

of Hospice Care, and the Comfort Care Concern Group, which offered community-based training and increased public awareness. Since 2007, the Hospital Authority and the Li Ka Shing Foundation's "Heart of Gold" Hospice Services Programme trained 800 volunteers as hospice service ambassadors. Although Hong Kong has a moderately-developed palliative care network, its level of community engagement is still below average, ranking 38th out of 80 according to the 2015 Quality of Death Index by The Economist Intelligence Unit [34]. This ranking indicates limited public awareness of EoLC services and a scarcity of volunteers available for EoLC in Hong Kong. The development of volunteerism in EoLC remains fragmented and lacks a systematic theoretical framework to guide its growth and integration.

The consolidation stage began in 2016 with the Jockey Club End-of-Life Community Care Project (JCECC) (http://www.JCECC.hk). Joining the global compassionate community movement, the Hong Kong Jockey Club Charities Trust has earmarked HKD $520 million (approximately USD $67 million) to initiate the project since 2016. This 10-year project is one of the first pioneer community-led EoLC projects in the Asia-Pacific region, which aims at developing a multi-institutional and cross-sectoral collaboration to improve the quality of EoLC in Hong Kong. Building on previous community EoLC interventions, the JCECC project in Hong Kong, guided by the five underpinning principles to facilitate the development of compassionate communities [35], adopts four main strategies (P3A strategies) to support people at end of life (**Figure 1**).

The P3A strategies—partnership, activation, action, and advocacy—offer a comprehensive framework to facilitate the development of compassionate communities for EoLC in Hong Kong. Through *partnerships* with universities, non-Government organizations (NGOs), hospitals, and local organizations, P3A harnesses a broad range of expertise and resources to create a robust support network. *Activation* focuses on enhancing capabilities through professional and volunteer training [2, 36], as well as raising awareness about EoLC, thereby equipping individuals and communities with the necessary skills and knowledge. In the *action* phase, through Integrated Community EoLC Support Teams, composed of professionals, volunteers, and community caregivers, deliver practical, physical, and psychosocial support to those in need, enhancing the overall well-being of patients and families [37]. Finally, *advocacy*

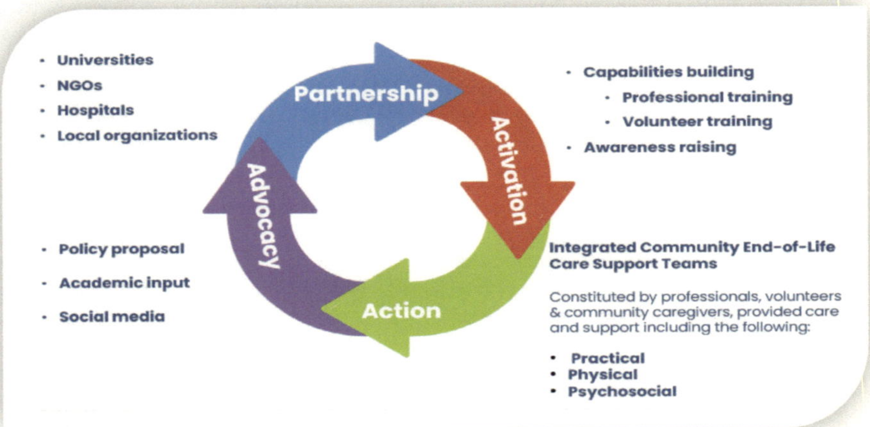

Figure 1.
P3A strategies.

involves policy proposals, academic input, and social media campaigns to influence public opinion and policy, ensuring that EoLC remains a priority on the social agenda. Together, these strategies create a synergistic approach that not only provides immediate care and support but also fosters a long-term, sustainable compassionate community in Hong Kong. In the following section, we focus on how we involve volunteers in this model to facilitate the development of compassionate communities in Hong Kong.

2. Facilitating compassionate community in Hong Kong

Since the JCECC project started in 2016, we have trained around 1500 volunteers by partnering with NGOs. Of 875 volunteers, we found that the majority (76.5%) were female and had attained a college education (72.2%). Employment status varied, with 30.9% working full-time, 16.5% working part-time, and the remaining participants being retired (19.9%), homemakers (8.9%), unemployed (10.3%), students (11.3%), or having other job conditions (2.3%). Regarding marital status, the two largest groups were single (44.8%), or married or cohabiting (45.6%). Additionally, two-thirds (59.4%) of the volunteers identified with a religion, whereas 40.6% did not. The age distribution showed that those aged 50 years or above constituted the largest group (48.3%). Although the age distribution differed from other studies [6, 10] (our sample being overall much younger), the demographic characteristics were otherwise similar to samples from different countries and regions.

Motivation played a key role in understanding why individuals volunteer [38, 39]. In our sample, we used the volunteer functions inventory to measure their motivations. The primary reasons for volunteering were altruistic purposes (value motivation) and the desire to gain or apply knowledge (understanding motivation). Other motivations included enhancement, career, protective, and social reasons. This finding aligns with other studies [10, 40], which have shown that most EoLC volunteers are driven by the desire to help others. We also employed the death anxiety s cale-15 items (5 Likert point) to measure their preparedness before training and found that their death anxiety level was a little bit higher than the average of the total score (Mean = 40.9, SD = 8.0, N = 542). Therefore, although participants interested in EoLC volunteering were motivated to help others, they needed to improve their knowledge of death-related topics, service capabilities, and skills. Thus it was clear that training for hospice and EoLC volunteers is essential [41–43].

However, currently, attention on EoLC volunteers has shifted from focusing solely on their demographic characteristics, personality traits, and motivations to also considering the sustainability of their service. There is limited information about the means by which volunteers strategically coordinate with existing in-service medical professionals, social workers, and third sector organizational partners in supporting a compassionate community approach to EoLC. Moreover, few volunteer-engaged compassionate community interventions were conducted with reference to theoretical capacity-building model for volunteers [44]. Therefore, this study aims to describe the evolution of a theory-driven volunteer partnerships with different key stakeholders in advocating compassionate Hong Kong communities, drawing insights from the JCECC Project. To this end, the volunteer training project adopted four strategies: partnership, capacity-building, nurturing leadership, and enabling coordination (**Figure 2**).

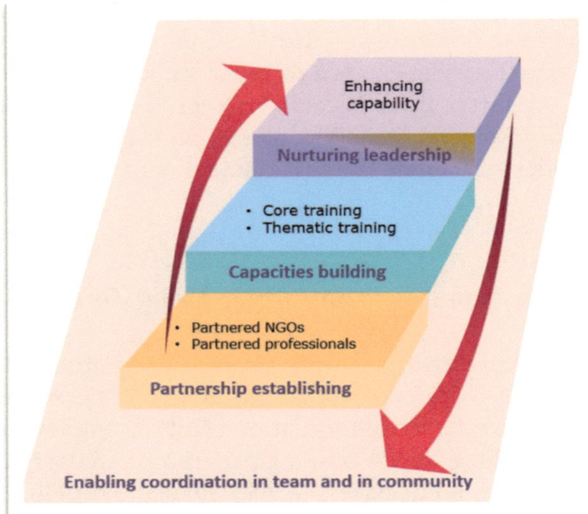
Enhancing capability
Nurturing leadership
• Core training
• Thematic training
Capacities building
• Partnered NGOs
• Partnered professionals
Partnership establishing
Enabling coordination in team and in community

Figure 2.
Four strategies for volunteering development.

2.1 Partnership

Partnership as a strategy to involve volunteers in EoLC services is exemplified through a collaborative approach at both organizational and team levels. At the organizational level, The University of Hong Kong has partnered with four non-profit government organizations—Hong Kong Society for Rehabilitation, Hope of Heaven Christian Services, S.K.H. Holy Carpenter Community Centre, and St. James' Settlement—to establish a cooperative mechanism for volunteer recruitment and training. Each organization sets different palliative care objectives tailored to their unique characteristics, while The University of Hong Kong is responsible for designing and providing the volunteer training programs. Beyond these four organizations, the university also reaches out to other local organizations, offering free courses to their volunteers, thereby fostering a community cooperation network.

On the team level, volunteers are integral members of the community integrated service teams, a key strategy developed by JCECC. They are primarily supervised by social workers, nurses, or care managers. Social workers adhere to the principle of cooperation by assessing the needs of the families they serve and then arranging appropriate services, including matching volunteers for patients and families, for home visits. Volunteers may also collaborate with nurses or other professional groups, working together to provide comprehensive care. As partners to other professionals, volunteers play an indispensable role within the team. But how do the volunteers understand their roles in the team? How do they work with other professionals? As a layman of EoLC, to be equipped to work and cooperate with other professionals in the team, volunteers need to be trained.

2.2 Capacity-building

We developed a theory-driven capacity-building model that was guided by an extensive review of the literature [44]. This model comprises four essential steps for competency development: motivational screening, core competence building, internships, and ongoing supervision and support. The specifics of these four steps have been detailed in other publication [44]. During the capacity-building phase, we establish three levels of training: core training, thematic training, and leadership training. The core training curriculum includes eight crucial modules: (1) Overarching values and knowledge in EoLC; (2) Volunteer roles and boundaries in EoLC; (3) Communication skills; (4) Psychosocial and spiritual care skills; (5) Symptom management and maintaining patient comfort and well-being; (6) EoL decision-making; (7) Bereavement care; and (8) Self-care and self-reflection. These modules are mandatory and equip volunteers with fundamental knowledge and skills in EoLC.

The foundational course spans four sessions, totaling 16 hours. However, during actual training, we observed a relatively-high dropout rate among EoLC volunteers [45, 46]. This may be linked to their motivations. As previously mentioned, some volunteers are primarily driven by a strong desire for knowledge, and they may withdraw from service upon completing the course. Additionally, volunteers often report forgetting many key points after the training, prompting them to retake the course in subsequent years. To address these issues, we have transitioned some knowledge-based content to an online self-learning platform. The JCECC volunteer online self-learning platform (https://volunteer.jcecc.hk/) has been available since 2023. This change allows instructors more time to design practice-related activities, such as role-playing and reflective discussions, to reinforce the knowledge acquired through online learning. The online self-learning platform provides a continuous learning environment for volunteers and introduces the general public to fundamental concepts of EoLC care and volunteer service, meeting the public's interest in EoLC topics.

The new training mode has shown notable initial outcomes. Firstly, it has broadened access to EoLC knowledge and skills for the general public. The previous training model was limited to volunteers selected by organizations, excluding those simply interested in learning about EoLC. Since the platform's launch in April 2023, it has achieved very encouraging results. By September 30, 2024, nearly 1440 users, including local participants, overseas Chinese, and learners from mainland China, have registered on the platform. Moreover, 340 individuals have participated in the instructor-led core training courses (through Zoom), indicating widespread interest and engagement in volunteer training program.

Secondly, data shows that participants who utilized the online self-learning platform in 2023 demonstrated significant improvements in EoLC capabilities compared to those who only attended instructor-led training courses. Although volunteers selected by organizations in 2022 started at a higher baseline, the percentage increase in capabilities among those who engaged with both the online platform and instructor-led courses was significantly higher ($p < 0.001$), particularly in basic concepts of EoLC, with improvement exceeding 40% (**Figure 3**).

In addition to the foundational training, volunteers are encouraged to further their skills by selecting advanced training topics that align with their interests and their perspectives on the demands of EoLC services. These advanced topics are delivered by thematic training and include telephone communication techniques, legal issues surrounding end-of-life, life review techniques, basic skills for managing family conflicts, and self-care strategies, among others. These specialized subjects enhance the volunteers' capabilities, providing them with the necessary expertise to contribute effectively within professional service teams. This approach ensures that volunteers are not only well-prepared to meet the diverse needs of EoLC, but are also empowered

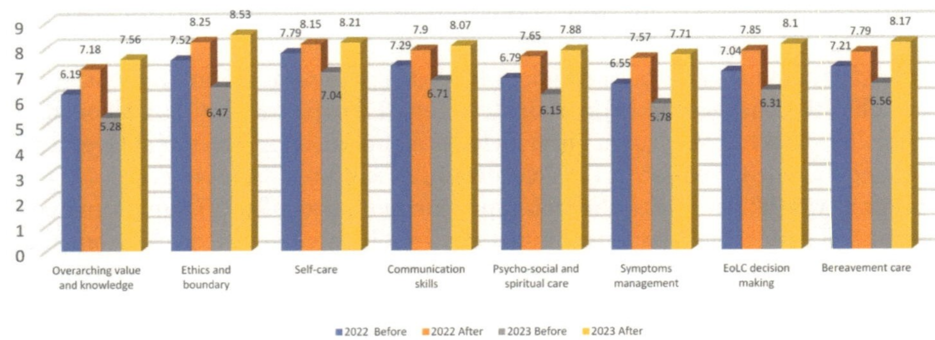

Figure 3.
Changes of competence after training in 2022 and 2023. Note: Before: before training; After: after training.

to engage more meaningfully in their volunteer role. This ultimately leads to successful functioning in multidisciplinary EoLC teams and communities.

2.3 Nurturing leadership

The Leadership Training Program is designed to provide participants with a platform to reflect on, and develop, their volunteer practice skills, as well as to acquire the necessary skills for peer support. The program consists of four workshops, with two components: "Leadership Skills Training" (taught by partner NGO staff) and "Core Competency Reflection" (taught by staff from the University of Hong Kong). "Leadership Skills Training" focuses on the skills needed for volunteers to fulfill their leadership roles. Topics include peer support, designing and implementing service activities, effective reporting techniques, and the ability to handle and resolve conflicts. On the other hand, "Core Competency Reflection" aims to enhance volunteers' personal abilities and growth. This segment covers self-awareness and self-care, emotional regulation, communication and expression skills, as well as motivation and commitment.

The Volunteer Leadership Training Program has been running consistently since it began in 2020. Over this time, it has nurtured 118 volunteer leaders. The majority have been women (n = 111; 71.2%). Most participants are aged 60 years or older (80.7%), with 47.3% being retirees and 15.5% being employed full-time, others are homemakers, students, and the like. Approximately two-thirds (67.9%) have religious affiliations. All these volunteer leaders have undergone foundational core training and were recommended by social workers based on their service abilities. Experienced volunteers from non-partner organizations can also apply for the leadership training through self-recommendation. Their applications are reviewed based on their volunteer service experience and EoLC background. Data shows that post-training, there is a significant improvement in volunteers' abilities to design activities, practice self-care, build teams, and communicate effectively. After training, these volunteers can contribute better in the EoLC team to mentor new volunteers and to increase their activity in EoLC activities in communities.

2.4 Enabling coordination

The training and management of EoLC volunteers in the community continues to have challenges. Despite the variety of volunteer programs for EoLC implemented in hospices and hospitals, there is little agreement on the specific skills needed by volunteers to effectively deliver EoLC in community settings [44]. Moreover, there is a high turnover rate of EoLC volunteers which highlights the importance of having comprehensive and effective EoLC volunteer management and support systems in place. This training is aimed at community-based individuals who are interested in providing EoLC, as well as institutions which currently involve volunteers in EoLC. Our training has four primary goals: (1) to help volunteer coordinators understand the value and significance of volunteers in EoLC services; (2) to equip coordinators with the skills needed to train volunteers to become qualified members of the multidisciplinary care team; (3) to motivate volunteers to collaborate effectively with professional healthcare workers; and (4) to sustain the engagement of EoLC volunteers, thereby facilitating the development of compassionate communities.

The training for EoLC volunteer coordinators is grounded in the SENS framework reference. This examines the capabilities and skills needed for the development and coordination of EoLC volunteer services from four perspectives: (1) Stimulating Shared Value, (2) Enabling Collective Action, (3) Nurturing an Integrated Team, and (4) Sustaining a Compassionate Community. Specific training topics include the value of EoLC volunteers, their role in the multidisciplinary care team, and the preparation required for involving volunteers in community-based EoLC service projects. The training thus covers the detailed processes of preparing, recruiting, selecting, training, and supporting EoLC volunteers.

Since 2020, the coordinator training program has trained 222 professionals, including social workers, nurses, health supporting workers, and other professionals. We also included experienced EoLC volunteers with more than 5 years' volunteering experiences in the training program, with the aim of upskilling them as volunteer coordinators to assist the professional health workers in the team. Post-training evaluations indicate a significant improvement in the coordinators' capacities in management skills, service coordination, and roles and boundaries setting.

Enhancing the capabilities of EoLC volunteers is a prerequisite for their effective participation in EoLC services, allowing them to integrate more seamlessly into care teams and exert even greater influences. By developing their leadership and team coordination skills, volunteers can expand the scope of their services, adopting a patient-centered approach that enables them to initiate community-based actions. This role is akin to the "connector" roles promoted in countries like Canada and Australia [22, 27]. Not only do they link patients with the community, but they also bridge isolated medical teams with community resources, thereby constructing a robust community support network for palliative care. This connector service has a significant impact on patients, families, and the community, as well as on the volunteers themselves. The impacts that we have identified through our findings are described below.

3. Impacts of volunteers on EoL care ecology

EoLC volunteering has profound impacts on the construction of compassionate communities, benefiting patients, families, volunteers, and society as a whole [20, 22]. Our study also highlights the impacts of volunteers on fostering compassionate communities (**Figure 4**).

For patients and families, volunteers provide essential practical support, psychosocial and spiritual care, and physical assistance, thereby enhancing quality of life

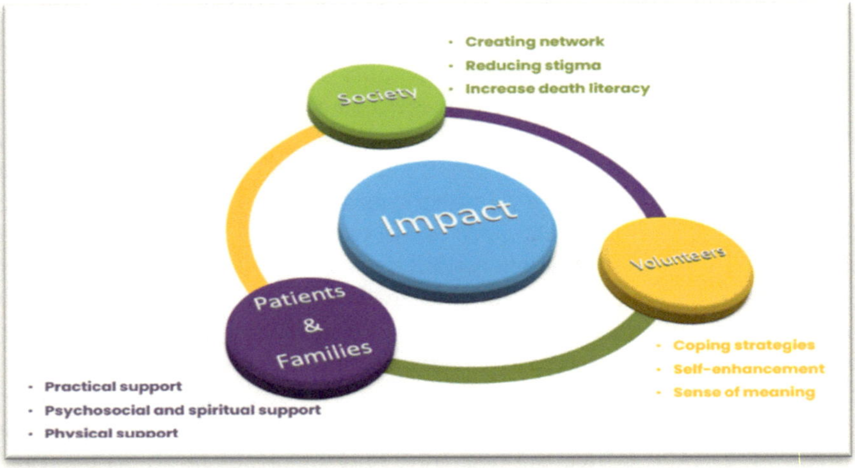

Figure 4.
Impacts on related holders.

in the final stages of life and ensuring that patients and families do not face these challenges alone. Volunteers themselves gain valuable coping strategies, opportunities for self-enhancement, and a deepened sense of meaning and purpose, which enriches their personal lives and fosters a compassionate outlook. On a societal level, EoLC volunteering helps create robust support networks that reduce the stigma associated with death and dying. By increasing death literacy, these efforts promote a more informed and accepting community that is better equipped to handle end-of-life issues with empathy and understanding. Collectively, these impacts contribute to the development of a compassionate community that values and supports its members throughout all stages of life.

3.1 Impact on patients

In this multidisciplinary care team, volunteers work closely with healthcare professionals to provide comprehensive support. Typically, social workers first assess patient and family situations before matching patients with suitable volunteers for home visits. According to service records, from 2019 to 2023, volunteers have contributed approximately 8700 hours of service, for 911 patients and their families. Their efforts have been guided by the 3-P need model, which addresses the *physical*, *psychological*, and *practical* needs of patients and their families. Specifically, they offer emotional support, social support, practical assistance, information support, spiritual support, and bereavement support. In the following section, three cases are presented to illustrate the many supports volunteers have provided for patients and families in the community. These cases can last up to 3 years.

3.1.1 Enhancing spiritual well-being

A year ago, Uncle Chung was diagnosed with lymphoma and nasopharyngeal cancer. His condition has been unstable, leading to multiple hospital admissions, and being fed through a nasogastric tube at times. Despite his illness, Uncle Chung, a devout Buddhist, remained concerned about the upkeep of the Buddhist altar in his home and the teachings of Buddhism. Due to his deteriorating health, he was unable to maintain the altar, resulting in a thick layer of dust accumulating on the statues, which deeply troubled him. Uncle Chung often lamented not being able to promote Buddhism and perform good deeds when he was healthier. He worried about the fate of the statues after his passing. Another of his wishes was to dine at the Chi Lin Nunnery, but living alone and with limited mobility, he struggled to take care of himself, let alone dine out. His spiritual distress led to increasing anxiety and depression, which further impacted on his deteriorating physical health.

The care team discussed Uncle Chung's situation and decided to arrange for volunteers to thoroughly clean his Buddhist altar. Seeing the bright and clean altar significantly improved Uncle Chung's mood, allowing him to chant Buddhist scriptures with a peaceful mind. One volunteer, who was knowledgeable about Buddhism, became Uncle Chung's spiritual companion, listening to his stories about his journey in becoming a Buddhist and adherence to its precepts. They discussed Buddhist teachings, scriptures, and ways to perform good deeds. Through their conversations, the volunteer discovered that "living like the Buddha" was a core belief for Uncle Chung, which he practiced by loving his family, community, and environment.

The care team then invited Uncle Chung to help with flag selling (note: philanthropic activity). His enthusiastic participation not only made him a fundraising star within the volunteer team but also fulfilled his wish to promote Buddhism. With his spiritual needs met, Uncle Chung's physical condition stabilized, and his spirits lifted. He is now actively planning with the care team to visit Chi Lin Nunnery for a vegetarian meal with his siblings and friends during the Lunar New Year. They also plan to discuss how to properly place the statues in his home. The dedicated efforts of the volunteers, coupled with the comprehensive support from the care team, played a crucial role in significantly improving Uncle Chung's spiritual and physical well-being. By addressing both his spiritual and practical needs, the volunteers not only enhanced his quality of life but also helped him achieve personal fulfillment and peace.

3.1.2 Reviving daily joy

Ninety-year-old Grandma Tong has been diagnosed with heart failure and breast cancer. While she faces her illnesses and the prospect of death with remarkable composure, her daily life limitations have become a significant burden. Hearing loss has rendered her unable to engage in conversations, and constant fatigue prevents her from managing household chores and taking care of her grandchildren. Her weakened limbs make her prone to falls, and a compromised immune system leaves her vulnerable to frequent pneumonia infections. This has led to a deep sense of depression and a feeling of emptiness and meaninglessness in her life.

The care team assessed that Grandma Tong's advanced illnesses were severely restricting her daily life and impacting her mood. They decided to invite volunteers to visit her at home and explore her interests and talents. During these visits, they discovered that Grandma Tong was an excellent cook with a particular talent for making traditional Chinese pastries. With the Mid-Autumn Festival approaching, the volunteers and care team, in coordination with Grandma Tong's family, planned a festive gathering. Volunteers accompanied Grandma Tong to the market to buy ingredients for making water chestnut cake. This opportunity to prepare food for her family again significantly lifted her spirits.

The volunteers later assisted Grandma Tong in making the pastries, which she then shared with other patients in the hospital. To pass on her culinary skills, Grandma

Tong began creating a recipe book for her family and the volunteers. This project gave her a renewed sense of purpose and transformed her life from being dominated by illness to one filled with meaningful activities and social engagement. The intervention by the volunteers played a crucial role in improving Grandma Tong's quality of life. By identifying and leveraging her cooking talent, they provided her with a sense of accomplishment and joy. This not only alleviated her feelings of emptiness but also strengthened her connections with her family and community. The volunteers' support in facilitating activities that Grandma Tong enjoyed had a substantial positive impact on her emotional well-being. It highlights the importance of addressing not just the physical but also the psychological and social needs of elderly patients, especially those with serious illnesses. By enriching her daily life and enabling her to share her skills, the volunteers helped transform Grandma Tong's experience from one of isolation and despair, to one of engagement and fulfillment.

3.1.3 Alleviating the physical pain

Seventy-year-old Mr. Lam has been living with Parkinson's disease for over a decade. His condition has progressively worsened over the past year, leading to significant deterioration in his lower limb strength and balance, causing frequent falls at home. Recently, his swallowing ability has declined, resulting in frequent choking episodes and subsequent pneumonia. These issues have led to recurrent hospital admissions. Mr. Lam, who was once active and enjoyed walking and socializing, now feels trapped at home, despondent, and awaiting the end of his life. Mrs. Lam, who is also elderly and suffers from arthritis, is physically weak and heavily burdened by the caregiving responsibilities, leading to stress-induced insomnia.

To help alleviate Mr. and Mrs. Lam's physical discomfort, the social worker invited a volunteer, who once was a registered nurse before retirement, to visit the Lams. She provided useful information to help Mr. and Mrs. Lam to understand their changing physical situations. They listened to the challenges faced by Mrs. Lam in caregiving and identified the causes of Mr. Lam's frequent falls. The volunteer provided several recommendations to improve their situation, including adjusting medication timings to better align with daily activities, installing grab bars in the bathroom and bedroom, using a shower chair, and switching to a walker.

Moreover, the professional volunteers taught Mr. and Mrs. Lam appropriate stretching and fall-prevention exercises suitable for Parkinson's patients. They also instructed Mrs. Lam on how to enhance Mr. Lam's protein intake to maintain muscle strength and demonstrated safer methods for daily activities, such as getting out of bed, walking, showering, and eating. To address his swallowing difficulties, they recommended using smaller spoons and feeding at a slower pace. They also guided Mrs. Lam on selecting and preparing appropriate foods to reduce the risk of choking. Since implementing these recommendations, Mr. Lam has not required any further hospital admissions. Community volunteers have also stepped in to accompany Mr. Lam on outings, significantly lifting his spirits. Mrs. Lam's caregiving burden has been alleviated, and she has been encouraged by her husband's improved condition. This newfound confidence has led her to venture outside more often. Additionally, their children are now more willing to spend time with their parents during holidays, taking them out for excursions. This strengthened family and community connection has substantially enhanced the quality of life for both Mr. and Mrs. Lam during this late stage of Mr. Lam's illness.

By making practical adjustments to their home environment and daily routines, Mr. and Mrs. Lam have significantly reduced the risk of falls and choking incidents, thereby preventing further hospitalizations. The physical exercises and dietary adjustments have helped maintain Mr. Lam's strength and overall health. The emotional support provided by community volunteers has rekindled Mr. Lam's interest in life, while the reduction in caregiving stress has improved Mrs. Lam's well-being. This case highlights the importance of a holistic approach that includes medical, practical, and emotional support to improve the quality of life for patients with advanced illnesses and their caregivers.

4. Summary

These stories highlight how EoLC volunteers can play a crucial role in fostering a compassionate and supportive community environment. By providing practical and emotional support to patients and their families, volunteers help to alleviate the heavy burden of caregiving. Their presence and assistance offer much-needed respite to caregivers, reducing stress and preventing burnout. This creates a sense of community where individuals feel supported and cared for, promoting a culture of empathy and mutual aid.

4.1 Impact on volunteers themselves

Our program evaluations have included annual focus groups and individual interviews, and we have followed up with volunteers and invited those willing to share their experiences. In total, 37 volunteers participated in focus groups in 2020 and 2021. Additionally, 14 volunteers took part in individual interviews in 2022 and 2023 to discuss their volunteering experiences.

Initial data analysis indicated that volunteering in EoLC offers profound and multifaceted benefits to the volunteers themselves. One key area of impact is in coping. Volunteers often develop enhanced coping mechanisms that help them manage stress and emotional challenges more effectively. The skills and knowledge gained through supporting patients and their families can be applied to their personal lives, enabling them to better support themselves, their families, and friends during difficult times. This experience fosters emotional resilience and equips volunteers with the tools to handle grief and loss more constructively.

Because that experience can contribute to my personal growth, helping others while also benefiting myself. Therefore, I wish to embrace more challenges to enrich my life. While I learn, I can also assist others. (volunteer1)

The takeaway from this experience is personal growth. When a close friend of mine recently passed away, I realized that my emotional management had improved. Although I was very sad, I was still able to help organize the memorial service, support their spouse, and listen to others who were also grieving. In the past, I might have cried a lot and felt like I could not accomplish anything. But now, I see that I have grown and changed. (volunteer2)

In addition to coping, volunteers experience significant self-enhancement and personal growth. The role encourages self-reflection, helping volunteers gain a deeper understanding of their values and motivations, which ultimately leads to personal improvement.

Interacting with patients and their families provides invaluable life lessons, fostering a greater appreciation for life and encouraging volunteers to cherish every moment. This experience also broadens their perspectives on life and death, contributing to a more profound sense of purpose and meaning.

When you are accompanying those people, you are not just serving them; you are also learning how to face death and life. This experience has made me cherish my own life more and better understand how to find meaning in it. The sense of purpose you gain is different from that of other volunteers. For most other volunteers, their beneficiaries are still alive, but what we need most is life itself, not money. (volunteer3)

I visited an elderly person, which gave me the opportunity to get to know them. During the process, I was able to help them conduct a life review. This was really wonderful; we took out all the photos at home, and I helped them write down their memories by hand. This was very meaningful. Both the elderly person and their family were very happy. Near the end of their life, they were able to find faith, and after they passed away, we gave the life review documentation to their family. It was a very joyful experience. This was a perfect experience. (volunteer4)

The fulfillment derived from being trusted, bringing happiness to others, and being appreciated for their efforts adds to the sense of value and meaning in their lives. Overall, EoLC volunteering not only benefits patients and their families but also significantly enriches the lives of the volunteers.

4.2 Impact on society

Volunteers often act as vital connectors between families facing end-of-life situations and the wider community. They facilitate communication and interaction, helping to reduce feelings of isolation and loneliness. By engaging with patients and their families, volunteers help integrate them into compassionate communities, ensuring that they remain connected and supported. This role is particularly important in creating a network of care that extends beyond the immediate family, fostering a sense of belonging and inclusion. What they do could be regarded as pioneering the development of a compassionate community, as one volunteer shared:

Actually, we are being deemed as an intermediary stage to start this process. Through this, we, as volunteers, become the first group—aside from professional personnel—to bring more attention to the conditions of elderly patients. This helps society to more calmly and readily accept matters related to death. So, I guess we can be considered a kind of, how should I put it, pioneer. (volunteer 5)

One of the significant impacts of EoLC volunteers is their contribution to reducing the stigma associated with death and dying. Through training, volunteers gain valuable insights into life and death education, which they share with their families, friends, and the broader community. By openly discussing topics related to death, they help to break down taboos and encourage a more open and honest dialog about end-of-life issues. This helps to normalize conversations about death, making it a less feared, and a more accepted part of life.

Volunteers also play a critical role in raising public awareness and knowledge about death and EoLC. By sharing their experiences and the information they have learned through training, they help to educate the community about the realities of terminal illnesses and the importance of compassionate care. This has increased awareness and empowered individuals to better support those facing end-of-life situations and encourages proactive planning and discussions about end-of-life wishes. As a result, society will become more informed and prepared to handle these challenging situations with sensitivity and care.

Ultimately, the impact of EoLC volunteers extends beyond individual patients and families to the broader society. By promoting a culture of compassion, reducing the stigma of death, and increasing death literacy, volunteers contribute to building a more empathetic and informed community. This leads to better support systems, enhanced quality of care for those at the end of life, and a society that values and respects the dignity of each individual, regardless of their stage in life.

5. Conclusion and implication

The introduction of volunteers into community-based EoLC has not only fostered public participation in EoLC issues but also heightened attention to the needs of terminally ill patients. Volunteers are the backbone of compassionate communities. The role of volunteers in the construction of compassionate communities extends far beyond the initial guidance provided by our project. Through the implementation of four key training strategies, volunteers have significantly enhanced their caregiving capabilities. These strategies have also improved their coordinating abilities in a multidisciplinary team and provided leadership training, enabling them to become proactive advocates for EoLC within their communities. This has paved the way for volunteers to effectively operate within the community, assuming roles such as connectors, supporters, and caregivers. Their involvement has had a profound impact on patients, helping them explore their meaning of life through activities like life reviews, and assisting them to fulfill their wishes. Moreover, volunteers facilitate the recovery of social connections for patients with their families, friends, and neighbors, often through the restoration of daily activities. This renewed sense of connectedness—spiritually, psychosocially, and physically—fosters a strong feeling of belonging for patients and their families within the community and the broader world.

Volunteers themselves derive mutual benefits from their participation. They experience a sense of reward from their contributions, undergo positive personal growth by confronting death, and gain deeper self-understanding. This involvement provides them with a sense of being valued and a clear purpose within the community, reinforcing their role as indispensable community assets. As pioneers in the construction of compassionate communities, volunteers promote life and death literacy within the community. They work to remove the stigma associated with death and cultivate a warm, open environment for discussing all aspects of life. Their efforts contribute to a more informed and accepting society, where discussions about death are no longer taboo but are embraced as part of the human experience.

With the involvement of volunteers in EoLC, a public health approach that relies on a close partnership between health services, community, and civic institutions is emerging as the optimal practice model. This collaboration exemplifies the effectiveness of combining professional health care with community-driven support, creating a robust framework for compassionate EoLC. This model has been endorsed as both feasible and acceptable in Hong Kong.

In conclusion, the involvement of volunteers in EoLC is transformative, benefiting not only patients and their families but also the volunteers themselves, and the community at large. Their contributions are essential in building compassionate communities that value empathy, support, and open discussions about life and death. This model of care serves as a testament to the power of community engagement in enhancing quality of life for all its members.

Acknowledgements

We thank our colleagues from the Jockey Club End-of-Life Community Care project team who provided insight and expertise that greatly assisted this study. We also thank our partners at the Hong Kong Society for Rehabilitation, Hope of Heaven Christian Services, S.K.H. Holy Carpenter Community Centre, and St. James' Settlement for their assistance with recruitment and training volunteers and providing valuable materials for data analysis of this study. We thank and salute those volunteers who participated in this project.

This work was supported by The Hong Kong Jockey Club Charities Trust.

Conflict of interest

The authors declare no conflict of interest.

Author details

Zhuyun Lin[1], Gloria Ka-Ming Chun[1], Felix Fung-Yu Mak[1], Victoria Ka-Ying Hui[1] and Vivian W.Q. Lou[1,2,3]*

1 Faculty of Social Science, The University of Hong Kong, Hong Kong, China

2 Sao Po Center on Aging, The University of Hong Kong, Hong Kong, China

3 Department of Social Work and Social Administration, The University of Hong Kong, Hong Kong, China

*Address all correspondence to: wlou@hku.hk

References

[1] Maresova P, Javanmardi E, Barakovic S, Barakovic Husic J, Tomsone S, Krejcar O, et al. Consequences of chronic diseases and other limitations associated with old age – A scoping review. BMC Public Health. 2019;**19**(1):1431

[2] Wong KTC, Chow AYM, Chan IKN. Effectiveness of educational programs on palliative and end-of-life care in promoting perceived competence among health and social care professionals. The American Journal of Hospice and Palliative Care. 2022;**39**(1):45-53

[3] Xiu D, Chow AYM, Chan IKN. Development and psychometric validation of a comprehensive end-of-life care competence scale: A study based on three-year surveys of health and social care professionals in Hong Kong. 2021;**19**(2):198-207

[4] World Health Organization. Palliative Care: Symptom Management and End-of-Life Care [Internet]. 2004. Available from: https://iris.who.int/bitstream/handle/10665/68535/WHO_CDS_IMAI_2004.4.pdf?sequence=4 [Accessed: December 2, 2024]

[5] Kelley LT, Coderre-Ball AM, Dalgarno N, McKeown S, Egan R. Continuing professional development for primary care providers in palliative and end-of-life care: A systematic review. Journal of Palliative Medicine. 2020;**23**(8):1104-1124

[6] Wong ELY, Kiang N, Chung RYN, Lau J, Chau PYK, Wong SYS, et al. Quality of palliative and end-of-life care in Hong Kong: Perspectives of healthcare providers. International Journal of Environmental Research and Public Health. 2020;**17**(14):5130

[7] Bijnsdorp F, Pasman H, Boot C, van Hooft S, van Staa A, Francke A. Profiles of family caregivers of patients at the end of life at home: A Q-methodological study into family caregiver' support needs. BMC Palliative Care. 2020;**19**(1):1-13

[8] Gardiner C, Barnes S. The impact of volunteer befriending services for older people at the end of life: Mechanisms supporting wellbeing. Progress In Palliative Care. 2016;**24**(3):159-164

[9] Pesut B, Duggleby W, Warner G, Fassbender K, Antifeau E, Hooper B, et al. Volunteer navigation partnerships: Piloting a compassionate community approach to early palliative care. BMC Palliative Care. 2018;**17**(1):2

[10] Morris S, Wilmot A, Hill M, Ockenden N, Payne S. A narrative literature review of the contribution of volunteers in end-of-life care services. Palliative Medicine. 2013;**27**(5):428-436

[11] Riffin C, Kenien C, Ghesquiere A, Dorime A, Villanueva C, Gardner D, et al. Community-based participatory research: Understanding a promising approach to addressing knowledge gaps in palliative care. Annals of Palliative Medicine. 2016;**5**(3):218-224

[12] Tilly C, Tilly C. Capitalist work and labor markets. In: Smelser N, Swedberg R, editors. Handbook of Economic Sociology. Princeton, NJ: Princeton University Press; 1994. pp. 283-313

[13] Vanderstichelen S. Palliative care volunteering: Pressing challenges in research. Palliative Medicine. 2022;**36**(4):564-566

[14] Fung FTW, Chan IKN, Lou VWQ. Building volunteer collaborative

leadership: An academic community partnership initiative. In: The Foundation of Community-Based End-of-Life Care in Hong Kong. 2019. pp. 249-267. Available from: https://foss.hku.hk/jcecc/en/innovation%E2%80%A7impact-the-foundation-of-community-based-eolc-in-hk/#1561606336794-fff98fce-0545 [Accessed: December 2, 2024]

[15] Walshe C, Algorta G, Dodd S, Hill M, Ockenden N, Payne S, et al. Protocol for the end-of-life social action study (ELSA): A randomised wait-list controlled trial and embedded qualitative case study evaluation assessing the causal impact of social action befriending services on end of life experience. BMC Palliative Care. 2016;**15**:1-9

[16] Morss S, Reder EA, McHale JM, Clayton TR, Silva C. Caring for patients in an inner-city home hospice: Challenges and rewards. Home Health Care Management and Practice. 2003;**15**(4):291-299

[17] Kellehear A. Compassionate Cities: Public Health and End-of-Life Care. London: Routledge; 2005

[18] Wegleitner K, Heimerl K, Kellehear A, editors. Compassionate Communities: Case Studies from Britain and Europe. 1st ed. South Oxfordshire: Routledge; 2016. Available from: https://www.taylorfrancis.com/books/9781317565079

[19] Ummel D, Vachon M, Guité-Verret A. Acknowledging bereavement, strengthening communities: Introducing an online compassionate community initiative for the recognition of pandemic grief. American Journal of Community Psychology. 2022;**69**(3-4):369-379

[20] Aoun SM, Abel J, Rumbold B, Cross K, Moore J, Skeers P, et al. The compassionate communities connectors model for end-of-life care: A community and health service partnership in Western Australia. Palliative Care. 2020;**14**:2632352420935130

[21] Horsfall D. Developing compassionate communities in Australia through collective caregiving: A qualitative study exploring network-centred care and the role of the end-of-life sector. Annals of Palliative Medicine. 2018;**7**(Suppl 2):S42-S51

[22] Noonan K, Rumbold B, Aoun SM. Compassionate community connectors: A distinct form of end-of-life volunteering. Progress in Palliative Care. 2023;**31**(1):1-10

[23] Vanderstichelen S, Dury S, De Gieter S, Van Droogenbroeck F, De Moortel D, Van Hove L, et al. Researching compassionate communities from an interdisciplinary perspective: The case of the compassionate communities center of expertise. The Gerontologist. 2022;**62**(10):1392-1401

[24] Liu CJ, Huang SJ, Wang SSC. Implementation of compassionate communities: The Taipei experience. Healthcare. Healthcare. 2022;**10**:1-10

[25] Paleri A, Numpeli M. The evolution of palliative care programmes in North Kerala. Indian Journal of Palliative Care. 2005;**11**(1):15-18

[26] Sallnow L, Kumar S, Numpeli M. Home-based palliative care in Kerala, India: The neighbourhood network in palliative care. Progress in Palliative Care. 2010;**18**(1):14-17

[27] Aoun SM, Richmond R, Noonan K, Gunton K, Rumbold B. 'The more you give, the better it is for you. You know the reward is greater than the effort': The compassionate communities connectors' experience. Palliative Care. 2022;**16**:26323524221139874

[28] Walshe C, Dodd S, Hill M, Ockenden N, Payne S, Preston N, et al. How effective are volunteers at supporting people in their last year of life? A pragmatic randomised wait-list trial in palliative care (ELSA). BMC Medicine. 2016;**14**:1-12

[29] Duggleby W, Pesut B, Warner G, Ruiz K, Nekolaichuk C, Ghosh S, et al. A feasibility study of a volunteer navigation program in the palliative context. American Journal of Hospice and Palliative Medicine. 2021;**38**(8):963-971

[30] Pesut B, Duggleby W, Warner G, Kervin E, Bruce P, Antifeau E, et al. Implementing volunteer-navigation for older persons with advanced chronic illness (Nav-CARE): A knowledge to action study. BMC Palliative Care. 2020;**19**(1):1-16

[31] Pesut B, Duggleby W, Warner G, Ghosh S, Bruce P, Dunlop R, et al. Scaling out a palliative compassionate community innovation: Nav-CARE. Palliative Care. 2022;**16**:26323524221095102

[32] Pesut B, Duggleby W, Warner G, Fassbender K, Antifeau E, Hooper B, et al. Volunteer navigation partnerships: Piloting a compassionate community approach to early palliative care. BMC Palliative Care. 2017;**17**:1-11

[33] Vocanec D, Loncarek K, Banadinovic M, Sovic S, Dzakula A. A qualitative study on the position and role of volunteers in integrated care-an example of palliative care in Croatia. International Journal of Environmental Research and Public Health. 2022;**19**(13):1-15

[34] The Economist Intelligence Unit. The 2015 Quality of Death Index: Ranking Palliative Care across the World. Lien Foundation [Internet]. 2015. Available from: https://impact.economist.com/perspectives/sites/default/files/2015%20EIU%20Quality%20of%20Death%20Index%20Oct%2029%20FINAL.pdf [Accessed: December 2, 2024]

[35] Australia, P. C. Compassionate Communities: An Implementation Guide for End-of-Life Care. 2018. Available from: https://ncq.org.au/wp-content/uploads/2018_NOUS_Compassionate-Communities_Implementation-Guide-for-End-of-Life-Care.pdf

[36] Takemura N, Fong DYT, Lin CC. Evaluating end-of-life care capacity building training for home care nurses. Nurse Education Today. 2022;**117**:105478

[37] Chow AYM, Fordjour GA, Lui JNM, Chan IKN, Zhang AY, Chan CLW. The physical and psychosocial outcomes of a psychosocial home-based end-of-life care intervention in Hong Kong. Journal of Palliative Care. 2023;**38**(4):481-489

[38] Clary EG, Snyder M, Ridge RD, Copeland J, Stukas AA, Haugen J, et al. Understanding and assessing the motivations of volunteers: A functional approach. Journal of Personality and Social Psychology. 1998;**74**(6):1516

[39] Claxton-Oldfield S, Wasylkiw L, Mark M, Claxton-Oldfield J. The inventory of motivations for hospice palliative care volunteerism: A tool for recruitment and retention. American Journal of Hospice and Palliative Medicine. 2011;**28**(1):35-43

[40] Nissim R, Emmerson D, O'Neill B, Marchington K, Draper H, Rodin G. Motivations, satisfaction, and fears of death and dying in residential hospice volunteers: A prospective longitudinal study. The American Journal of Hospice and Palliative Care. 2016;**33**(4):335-339

[41] Claxton-Oldfield S, Hicks R, Claxton-Oldfield J. A pilot study

evaluating the effectiveness of a training module designed to improve hospice palliative care volunteers' ability to deal with unusual end-of-life phenomena. Omega (Westport). 2022;**85**(1):75-87

[42] McGlinchey T, Mason S, Smeding R, Goosensen A, Ruiz-Torreras I, Haugen D, et al. ILIVE project volunteer study. Developing international consensus for a European core curriculum for hospital end-of-life-care volunteer services, to train volunteers to support patients in the last weeks of life: A Delphi study. Palliative Medicine. 2022;**36**(4):652-670

[43] Söderhamn U, Flateland S, Fensli M, Skaar R. To be a trained and supported volunteer in palliative care - A phenomenological study. BMC Palliative Care. 2017;**16**(1):18

[44] Wang Q, Chan IKW, Lou VWQ. Effectiveness of a holistic capacity-building program for volunteers in community-based end-of-life care. Research on Social Work Practice. 2020;**30**(4):408-421

[45] Hayslip B, Sethi A, Pinson MW, Carpenter C. Predicting attrition among hospice volunteers. Omega: Journal of Death and Dying. 2021;**84**(1):289-306

[46] Claxton-Oldfield S, Claxton-Oldfield J. Keeping hospice palliative care volunteers on board: Dealing with issues of volunteer attrition, stress, and retention. Indian Journal of Palliative Care. 2008;**14**(1):30-37

Chapter 10

Perspective Chapter: Home-Based Palliative Care – Is there a Future?

Mateja Lopuh

Abstract

Home-based or community palliative care is desired by the majority of patients facing an incurable disease. The organization of such care presents a huge burden for health systems and communities as well as for the families and other informal caregivers who are part of the care. Despite patients' wishes, such care is sometimes not feasible, and the patients are being referred to different institutions. Balancing between wishes and possibilities is a challenge for different providers of home care, which spans through the continuum of the disease and may in the end result in referring the patient to institutionalized care, therefore questioning the cost-effectiveness of such care. Integrating such care into the health system requires recognition of its meaning and benefit that it may bring as well as reducing the burden of patients' care on other structures in the health care system.

Keywords: home-based palliative care, community care, informal caregivers, end of life, bereavement

1. Introduction

Better quality of life, better work conditions, and improvements in medical treatment have raised the life expectancy bar to a higher level. People live longer and expect a good quality of life for its entire length. Many are not spared from different diseases, which are not curable despite all the technological advances. Living with a disease places a burden on the patient, influences daily activities, limits life goals, and requires a lot of adjustments. The patient's social network is also included, supporting him through the disease trajectory and providing care.

Ninety percent of the final year is spent at home, no matter where the patient eventually dies [1]. The manner in which people die has been changing over the last generations. Dying is often prolonged and has primarily become the domain of the healthcare system [2, 3].

Most countries have data that home setting is the preferred place of care and death for the majority of people. Many caregivers support that idea, but the willingness to care declines with symptom burden and increased dependency of the patients [4].

In general opinion, home is a known place, although the living conditions are many times poor. Home should be a safe place for all, but sometimes there is terror and family violence, which is discovered only after health services visit the patient at home. It is very important to include all dimensions of patients' lives when deciding about the best place of care and death. It is also of utmost importance that health and social workers who attend to the patient and the family feel safe at work. It is not rare nowadays that domestic violence outreaches the home walls and is projected toward professionals who provide care.

Home-based palliative care means organization of care in the home environment of the patient. It is provided by community health programs and encompasses care in the home, hospice programs, or residential senior homes [5]. Many meta-analyses have been published with no conclusive results about health-related outcomes.

It is expected that the demand for service will expand due to changes in disease prevalence and prolonged duration of illness. On the other hand, it will be challenged by decreased assumption of caregivers' roles by family. Current models of palliative care might not be effective anymore, as the manpower to support their work is not sufficient in many countries. From an economic point of view, the stakeholders might not be satisfied with the little change in medical outcomes achieved by such services and the investments needed for their activity [5, 6].

Palliative care services should respond to the needs of the patient and caregivers. Patients ought to be as free of symptoms as possible and feel secure and supported. They need proactive planning along the expected trajectory of the disease. Caregivers need time to ask questions, to talk, to relieve their anxiety, and to be able to better understand the course of illness and the burden it brings along. Their bereavement process begins while adapting their lives to the needs of the patient. The most common reason for their breakdown is sleep deprivation and calls for simultaneous assessment of symptoms in the patient and in the caregiver [7].

The burden of care, constant availability, and the expectation to always properly address the needs of the patient and the caregiver put enormous pressure on the palliative care providers [8]. They should be more supported throughout their work and have a possibility to ventilate their emotions in a safe environment.

2. Definition of palliative care

Palliative care was initially and historically focused on alleviating the relief of suffering at the end of life. It was focused largely on patients with cancer. It has now developed into the care that is integrated into the treatment of all life-threatening health conditions and implemented early in the disease trajectory. Existing research suggests that PC is both effective in reducing symptom burden and improving quality of life, cost-effective, and synonymous with quality of care [9].

In 1990, WHO published a definition of palliative care and in 1998, a specific one for children. The WHO definition was revised in 2002 [10, 11]. It limits PC to problems associated with life-threatening illnesses, rather than the burdensome experience of patients with severe and frequently multiple chronic conditions. The range and severity of potential PC needs may be more relevant indicators of need for these patients than prognosis alone.

2.1 The Lancet Commission on global access to palliative care and pain relief

The Lancet Commission identified the need to review and revise the definition of PC.

New definition:

PC is the active holistic care of individuals across all ages with SHS (suffering is health-related when it is associated with illness or injury of any kind). Health-related suffering is serious when it cannot be relieved without medical intervention and when it compromises physical, social, or spiritual well being because of severe illness (severe illness is a condition that carries a high risk of mortality, negatively impacts quality of life and daily function, and/or is burdensome in symptoms, treatments, or caregivers' stress), and especially for those near the end of life. It aims to improve the quality of life of patients, their families, and their caregivers [12, 13].

3. Models of palliative care

The proportion of patients supported at home until death, if this is their preference, remains an important performance indicator for many communities' palliative care programs. Although stating home as their preference, the majority of patients face the last days of their lives in hospitals or similar facilities.

Many studies have tried to develop a tool that would enable easy identification of the patients who could be cared for at home and would also die at home. Although patients state such care as their preference, it is well known that preferences change with time and the progression of the disease. Even those with a good and supportive social network change their minds if they experience that care becoming a burden for their caregivers and believe that the caregivers do not have enough support.

Home care programs often face reluctance from caregivers who might regard the presence of professionals as intrusive. Palliative care programs are introduced too late in the course of the disease when both the patient and caregiver are too tired and exhausted and cannot cope any longer. Symptom burden also increases, and if not treated well from its onset, sleep deprivation of the caregiver can play an important role in deciding to admit the patient to the hospital.

It is aimed that home-based models of care should be intensive, sustained, and coordinated; services should not overlap. They should offer constant support to caregivers and aim to follow patients' wishes to be cared for and to die at home.

Community-based palliative care, or home-based palliative care, provides in-person visits, equipment supplies, and telephone support to patients. Care may be led by a specialist palliative care physician, nurse, or family doctor and usually occurs in a multidisciplinary team. It was shown that while any home-based medical care decreased the likelihood of dying in the hospital, those patients who received care from non-palliatively trained physicians were 12% more likely to die in the hospital [12–17]. Different models of palliative care in community are presented below.

3.1 Specialist palliative care physician-led multidisciplinary approach

Provided care 24/7, regular visits, and telephone support.

Compared with standard care.

This resulted in increased home deaths, patient and carer satisfaction, decreased hospital days, and decreased health care costs.

3.2 Family doctor and community nurse

Additional training in palliative care, supported by a specialist palliative care team for advice and visits.

Compared with standard palliative care.
More likely to die at home, but time at home and hospitalizations are similar.

3.3 Nurse-led palliative care program

Round-the-clock support in the last 2 weeks, low inclusion rate of the admissible patients.

No difference.

Although the studies are few and it is difficult to draw conclusions, most authors would agree that patients and caregivers appreciate continuity, coordination, and ongoing relationships with their primary care team or specialist provider. It is the orchestration of the services and the amount of practical and communication skills that increase the likelihood of the patient dying at home if so preferred. One could speculate that hospital-founded specialist palliative care teams in home settings would act as gatekeepers of the hospital and aim more to keep the patient at home.

There are several other models for providing specialist palliative care in the community setting, found in the literature.

a. Consultation model: Specialist advice is provided on assessment and treatment of symptoms and communication about goals of care and support. Advice is provided without necessarily assuming primary responsibility for care.

b. Liason model: Combines the education of patients after discharge with educational outreach and clinical support for primary care physicians.

c. Pop-up model: Developing a pop-up palliative service according to demand, using local resources and services.

Special attention should be given to providing palliative care in residential homes. Residential homes are considered home settings for their dwellers. Medical and nursing care is provided on-site. Therefore, the residents are rarely referred to specialist palliative care services. They are more likely to have poor symptom control, to be referred for admission more frequently, to have inadequate advance care planning, and more often, the families are not satisfied with end-of-life care. The most common missing elements of effective palliative support are

- Identifying residents who could benefit from referral to a specialist palliative provider
- Poorly educated staff, no feedback on performance
- No systematic symptom control strategies

Patients who circulate between care settings (community, residential care, and hospital) need to be given special attention. Important information might be lost through transition. The importance of supporting transitions is especially underscored in dementia. Health professionals in acute care may lack information if a palliative approach is appropriate and begin with inappropriate treatment, which would lead to prolongation of life with a massive negative effect on the quality of life [5, 8].

3.4 Most common barriers to dying at home

Death in a hospital is more likely if patients are poor, elderly, have no caregivers, are female, or have a long illness. The reasons for hospital admissions are mostly unresolved symptom control, a breakdown in the provision of home care services, and a lack of support for caregivers. Also, an important barrier is the reluctance of the primary health team to include a patient in specialist services.

One of the strong determinants for not being able to die at home is to be living alone. This group in the population will be increasing in time and present a bigger challenge for providers of home care [18].

Other factors can be divided into [18]:

a. Factors related to illness: missed transition to palliative care

b. Individual factors: patient's preference, personal investment, social factors, and ethnicity

c. Environmental factors: use of home care, social support, and macrosocial factors

4. Assessment of efficacy

When introducing new models of care, it is important to be able to show their efficacy or benefits for the unit of care, which in palliative care are the patient and his/her proxies. Community care is organized with the purpose of following patients' preferences for the place of death. It should be associated with a greater number of deaths in a home setting, but it is not yet clear if symptom control is adequate, what burden is placed upon caregivers, and if it is cost-effective.

Future research in this area should also include the health system's ability to provide such services due to the increasing lack of staff in all settings.

5. Supporting caregivers

Home support in any organizational structure highly depends on the involvement of informal caregivers, people close to the patient, who will support the patient through the disease trajectory. There are many challenges experienced by the caregivers. These can be divided into several categories:

a. Practical needs: It is essential to have access to professional support 24/7; only such continuity of care enables the caregivers to build trust with healthcare professionals. Some prioritize and find it reassuring if there is a constant person assigned to the patient and family.

b. Emotional and psychosocial needs: Transition from a family role to a carer's role, putting their lives on hold to be able to take care of their loved ones. Along the disease trajectory, patients change their attitude toward their caregivers and change their mood from being grateful to anger, sometimes even hate.

c. Spiritual needs: Caregivers are prompted to reexamine their life priorities; for some, it is a privilege but also a terrible burden, a duty, an obligation required due to life circumstances (not being able to pay for formal care, not being able to move out of the house, etc.).

d. Informational needs: Timely access to relevant information about symptom control.

One of the most important physical consequences of caregivers' health is sleep deprivation, causing increased fatigue, poor tolerance, and lower resilience. When it is decided that a home setting is the place of care for the patient and the carer, it is important to draw a trajectory of disease burden and adjustment that are needed in the carer's life. Proper planning and addressing the caregivers' needs result in a trustful relationship.

It is of utmost importance to get formal care when caring becomes too hard for informal caregivers.

All health strategies should support care at home, given by informal caregivers but not as compensation for deficiencies in formal palliative home care services [19–21].

6. Last days of life at home

The last days of life at home can be very stressful, as most of the caregivers go through this phase in life for the first time. It is emotionally and physically demanding. On the other hand, it can also be very rewarding for those who really wish to help. A lot of patients' dignity and values are at stake. Increasing physical fatigue and dependence on other people's help in eating, drinking, dressing, bathing, and other daily life activities can cause tension between caregivers and the patient.

Proper guidance and the ability to talk to someone build self-confidence. Palliative professionals should explain the symptoms the patient is likely to experience. Experience shows that although caregivers get a lot of information, they perceive missed opportunities as well for healthcare professionals to effectively collaborate with them for palliative care.

Caregivers should expect physical and cognitive changes in the patient. Cognitive decline is, for many, a sign that they are losing their beloved one. Sometimes this decline prompts the caregiver to call emergency services, thinking that the patient would no longer care about not being at home. It is very important to discuss such situations with a palliative care team.

Very often there are discussions about hydration and nutrition. Patients often become less interested in food and drink. They should be offered small sips of water and small portions of food they like most. Caregivers should be reassured that the patients do not feel hungry and they do not need too much to drink. If pressed to eat and drink, they could feel uncomfortable. In spite of all efforts by the palliative team, some family members remain frightened that the patient will die of hunger and thirst. In many countries, this fear has a broader background and could lead to being accused of negligence if not offering food and drink. Patients are sometimes pushed to receive artificial feeding tubes. If such tendencies are pursued by a team, special attention should be given, and caregivers' fears should be addressed in a family meeting.

Many physical symptoms tend to decline when the patient is approaching death. Some caregivers can be confused with the medications as they are needed less and when the patient is no longer able to swallow. Palliative care teams should respond promptly to the changes to allow adequate symptom control. The route of drug administration should be adjusted. Sometimes when a patient is experiencing multiple symptoms, subcutaneous elastomeric balloon pumps are used.

Care in the last days is focused on little but important things such as gentle massage, mouth care, aromatherapy, and relaxing music. Visiting hours should be reduced.

Caregivers should be given written instructions about what to do at the time of death. They should feel free to call in an uncertain situation about the death. Sometimes the palliative team can help in arranging the death certificate.

Palliative care providers should also hand out contact numbers for the bereavement period. Caregivers who were identified during the palliative care process as the ones who might need support in the bereavement phase should be provided with advice on how to cope before death [22–27].

7. Support for the care team

Palliative care teams usually consist of dedicated professionals who put more than just work into their care. They have a lot of empathy and good communication skills and are willing to understand and talk with the caregivers, who very often have greater needs than the patient itself. Specialist palliative care providers in home-based palliative care should provide support 24/7 in-home visits and telephone support. It is a challenging requirement nowadays, as there is a big shortage of staff. Few countries can follow the requirement; other countries will find approximation models, often combining specialist and basic palliative care, consultation models, and pop-up models.

Members of the teams should have the possibility of psychological support, intervisions, and supervision. Team-building meetings are great opportunities to ventilate, redefine goals, and reconnect. Often difficult home situations in some patients and their remarks to members of the team can put tension on team dynamics. Evaluation talks are very needed [28].

Team leaders should pay special attention to the needs of team members. There should be a great amount of trust between them.

Characteristics of a healthy palliative care team [28]:

- Strong leadership
- Clear roles and responsibilities
- Team well-being: positive relationship

8. Conclusion

The best palliative care should be accessible to all who need it. It should be tailored to patients'needs; the unit of care should include the caregivers providing care for the patient. Specialist palliative care should be introduced in a timely manner to patients with complex needs and should be available as a consultation model for basic palliative care providers. Population-based models of palliative care should be flexible to accommodate the rapidly changing needs of the population [5, 29]. It is highly likely that in the future different pop-up models would be more effective in providing care when needed than fixed structures. The future does not look bright in the sense of supporting informal caregivers, therefore putting home-based palliative care on the edge and forcing it to come up with new ideas.

Author details

Mateja Lopuh
General Hospital Jesenice, Slovenia

*Address all correspondence to: mateja.lopuh@gmail.com

References

[1] Thomas K. Community palliative care. In: Fallon M, Hanks G, editors. ABC Palliative Care. Blackwell Publishing; 2006. pp. 68-73. Available from: https://goldstandardsframework.org.uk/cd-content/uploads/files/Library,%20Tools%20%26%20resources/ABC%20Palliative%20Care.pdf [Accessed: March 21, 2025]

[2] Thomas K, Gray SM. Population-based, person-centred end-of-life care: Time for a rethink. The British Journal of General Practice. 2018;**68**(668):116-117

[3] Gomas J-M. Palliative care at home: A reality or mission impossible? Palliative Medicine. 1993;7:45-59

[4] Higginson IJ, Sen-Gupta GJ. Place of care in advanced cancer: A qualitative systematic literature review of patient preferences. Journal of Palliative Medicine. 2000;**3**(3):287-300

[5] Stokes C, Good P. Community palliative care: What are the best models? Current Treatment Options in Oncology. 2024;**25**(12):1550-1555

[6] Gomes B, Calanzani N, Curiale V, McCrone P, Higginson IJ. Effectiveness and cost-effectiveness of home palliative care services for adults with advanced illness and their caregivers. Cochrane Database of Systematic Reviews. 2013;**2013**:12-31

[7] King N, Bell D, Thomas K. Family carers' experiences of out-of-hours community palliative care: A qualitative study. International Journal of Palliative Nursing. 2004;**10**(2):76-83

[8] Luckett T, Phillips J, Agar M, Virdun C, Green A, Davidson PM. Elements of effective palliative care models: A rapid review. BMC Health Services Research. 2014;**14**:136

[9] World Health Assembly. Strengthening of Palliative Care as a Component of Comprehensive Care within the Continuum of Care. 2014. Available from http://apps.who.int/gb/ebwha/pdf_files/WHA67/A67_R19-en.pdf [Accessed: February 18, 2025]

[10] World Health Organization. Cancer Pain Relief and Palliative Care. Report of a WHO Expert Committee. Geneva: World Health Organization; 1990

[11] World Health Organization. National Cancer Control Programmes. Policies and Managerial Guidelines. 2nd ed. Geneva: World Health Organization; 2002

[12] Radbruch L, De Lima L, Knaul F, Wenk R, Ali Z, Bhatnaghar S, et al. Redefining palliative care-a new consensus-based definition. Journal of Pain and Symptom Management. 2020;**60**(4):754-764

[13] Knaul FM, Farmer PE, Krakauer EL, et al. Alleviating the access abyss in palliative care and pain relief—An imperative of universal health coverage: The lancet commission report. Lancet. 2018;**391**:1391-1454

[14] Murray SA, Kendall M, Mitchell G, et al. Palliative care from diagnosis to death. BMJ. 2017;**356**:j878

[15] Gomez-Batiste X, Connor S. Building Integrated Palliative Care Programs and Services. Barcelona: Liberdúplex; 2017

[16] Shepperd S, Gonçalves-Bradley DC, Straus SE, Wee B. Hospital at home:

Home-based end-of-life care. Cochrane Database of Systematic Reviews. 2021;**3**(3):8-14

[17] Riolfi M, Buja A, Zanardo C, Marangon CF, Manno P, Baldo V. Effectiveness of palliative home-care services in reducing hospital admissions and determinants of hospitalization for terminally ill patients followed up by a palliative home-care team: A retrospective cohort study. Palliative Medicine. 2014;**28**(5):403-411

[18] Gomes B, Higginson IJ. Factors influencing death at home in terminally ill patients with cancer: Systematic review. BMJ. 2006;**332**(7540):515-521

[19] Mohammed S, Swami N, Pope A, Rodin G, Hannon B, Nissim R, et al. "I didn't want to be in charge and yet I was": Bereaved caregivers' accounts of providing home care for family members with advanced cancer. Psycho-Oncology. 2018;**27**(4):1229-1236

[20] Bee PE, Barnes P, Luker KA. A systematic review of informal caregivers' needs in providing home-based end-of-life care to people with cancer. Journal of Clinical Nursing. 2009;**18**(10):1379-1393

[21] Vermorgen M, Vandenbogaerde I, Van Audenhove C, Hudson P, Deliens L, Cohen J, et al. Are family carers part of the care team providing end-of-life care? A qualitative interview study on the collaboration between family and professional carers. Palliative Medicine. 2021;**35**(1):109-119

[22] Jordhøy MS, Fayers P, Saltnes T, Ahlner-Elmqvist M, Jannert M, Kaasa S. A palliative-care intervention and death at home: A cluster randomised trial. Lancet. 2000;**356**(9233):888-893

[23] Brumley R, Enguidanos S, Jamison P, Seitz R, Morgenstern N, Saito S, et al. Increased satisfaction with care and lower costs: Results of a randomized trial of in-home palliative care. Journal of the American Geriatrics Society. 2007;**55**(7):993-1000

[24] Hughes SL, Cummings J, Weaver F, Manheim L, Braun B, Conrad K. A randomized trial of the cost effectiveness of VA hospital-based home care for the terminally ill. Health Services Research. 1992;**26**(6):801-817

[25] Grande GE, Todd CJ, Barclay SI, Farquhar MC. A randomized controlled trial of a hospital at home service for the terminally ill. Palliative Medicine. 2000;**14**(5):375-385

[26] Grande GE, Todd CJ, Barclay SI, Farquhar MC. Does hospital at home for palliative care facilitate death at home? Randomised controlled trial. BMJ. 1999;**319**(7223):1472-1475

[27] Caring for someone in their last days and hours. 25 Nov 2022. Available from: https://www.mariecurie.org.uk/professionals/palliative-care-knowledge-zone/last-days-and-hours

[28] Ragsdale L, Ullrich CK, Thienprayoon R, Miller EG, Humphrey L, Williams CSP, et al. Leading a palliative care team through times of growth and change. Journal of Palliative Medicine. Nov 2024;**27**(11):1439-1449

[29] Roberts B, Robertson M, Ojukwu EI, Wu DS. Home based palliative care: Known benefits and future directions. Current Geriatrics Reports. 2021;**10**(4):141-147

Section 4

Innovation

Chapter 11

Perspective Chapter: Sparsh Hospice – A Humanistic Bio-Psycho-Social Model of Compassionate, No-Cost Palliative Care

Padma Sesha Sarada Lingaraju

Abstract

Sparsh Hospice, an 82-bed facility in Hyderabad, India, provides free, high-quality palliative care for patients facing serious illnesses, particularly those from economically disadvantaged backgrounds. Founded in 2011 as a 12-bed unit, it has expanded into a comprehensive care centre, integrating inpatient, outpatient, and home care services. A fleet of well-equipped vans ensures accessible home-based care, allowing patients to receive support in familiar surroundings. Following a bio-psycho-social model, Sparsh addresses physical, emotional, social, and spiritual well-being, offering services beyond medical treatment. Families receive nutritional assistance, bereavement support, funeral aid, and connections to non-profits for livelihood and children's education. The hospice actively promotes awareness and education, integrating palliative care into medical curricula and conducting rural outreach programs. Volunteers contribute to patient comfort through music, art, and engagement, fostering a compassionate community that enhances the quality of life. Sparsh Hospice goes beyond patient care, advocating for palliative care accessibility and acceptance. It works closely with schools, universities, and healthcare institutions to cultivate empathy and early awareness among future healthcare providers. Community support plays a crucial role in its sustainability, enabling it to function as a non-commercialised model. Through collaboration and outreach, Sparsh bridges healthcare gaps, ensuring that patients receive dignified, compassionate care at no cost. As a leader in humanistic palliative care, Sparsh continues to provide holistic support to those in need, offering not just medical relief but also emotional and social security to patients and families.

Keywords: hospice, palliative care, India, no-cost care, holistic care

1. Introduction

Sparsh Hospice, a stand-alone hospice care facility, was established to address the glaring gap in palliative care accessibility and acceptance in India, where less than 10% of individuals in need receive the care, they deserve. The organisation was founded with the firm belief that pain management and dignity in death are fundamental human rights. Sparsh Hospice has not only pioneered efforts to make palliative care available but has also worked tirelessly to shift societal perceptions, making the acceptance of palliative care an integral part of its mission. With the mission of health for all, Aarogyasri is the health initiative of the State Government of Telangana. Its mission is to provide quality healthcare to communities with low resources. It provides financial assistance to meet the needs of it communities [1]. With such support, Sparsh is able to care for patients and families with serious illness, taking an approach that is rooted in the philosophy that compassionate care should transcend barriers of socioeconomic status, illness type, or cultural stigma, offering support to anyone who needs it.

What sets Sparsh Hospice apart is its development as a humanistic, non-profit model of care. It embraces the philosophy that every individual deserves relief from suffering and support in their journey, regardless of their background. This approach is inclusive, looking beyond cancer and extending care to patients with a range of serious ailments. By addressing physical, emotional, and spiritual needs, Sparsh Hospice has become a sanctuary for those seeking compassionate end-of-life care or management of chronic conditions.

Since its inception in 2011 as a modest 12-bedded facility, Sparsh Hospice has grown into a state-of-the-art 82-bedded inpatient hospice, reflecting its commitment to meeting the increasing demand for high-quality, compassionate care. Alongside its inpatient services, the organisation has developed extensive home care programs, making care accessible to patients in rural and interior parts of Telangana and neighbouring states. To further its reach, Sparsh Hospice has also introduced outpatient services, ensuring that patients who cannot access its inpatient facility or home care programs still receive essential palliative support.

A significant milestone in Sparsh Hospice's journey is its recent empanelment under the *Rajiv Aarogyasri (Telangana- state) Government Healthcare Insurance Scheme*, making it the first stand-alone hospice in India to achieve this recognition. This empanelment has been a step towards increasing its reach and strengthening sustainability. However, Sparsh Hospice remains deeply committed to its founding philosophy, reaffirming its dedication to serving individuals even outside the purview of government reimbursement schemes. The organisation espouses the belief in extending care to all those in need, irrespective of their inclusion in healthcare policies, ensuring that no one is left behind [2].

Beyond patient care, Sparsh Hospice has delved deeply into initiatives that create lasting change. It incorporates training and sensitisation programs into school curriculums, fostering a culture of empathy and understanding in younger generations. These efforts aim to create a more compassionate society that recognises the importance of supporting individuals and families during the most challenging phases of life.

Over the past 13 years, Sparsh Hospice has grown into a beacon of hope, not only for patients and families but also for society at large. Its commitment to advocacy, education, and systemic transformation has made it more than just a care provider; it has become a movement that reshapes how palliative care is perceived and practised in the Indian context.

Before delving into the specifics of Sparsh Hospice's programs and initiatives, including its inpatient services, home care programs, outpatient services, and advocacy efforts, it is important to understand how these multifaceted efforts continue

DOI: http://dx.doi.org/10.5772/intechopen.1009161

to address the evolving needs of patients and families, both within and outside the purview of reimbursement schemes and why this type of care is essential.

2. Expanding the scope of palliative care

In many parts of the world, including India, there is a common misconception that palliative care and hospice care are exclusively meant for terminally ill cancer patients [3]. Sparsh Hospice has worked diligently to address this misunderstanding, creating awareness about the distinction between *palliative care* and *hospice care*. Palliative care is designed for patients undergoing active treatment for serious illnesses, focusing on symptom management, pain relief, and enhancing the quality of life [4]. Hospice care, on the other hand, is intended for terminal patients, ensuring dignity, comfort, and support during the final stages of life [5].

Sparsh Hospice has expanded the scope of palliative care beyond traditional boundaries. It actively serves patients suffering from a variety of serious health-related issues, including neurodegenerative diseases, multi-organ failures, and other chronic conditions that significantly affect their quality of life. By addressing debilitating symptoms such as pain, breathlessness, and fatigue, the organisation ensures that patients receive comprehensive care tailored to their specific needs. This holistic approach does not stop at the patient; it also provides a robust support system for families, recognising the critical role they play in the patient's journey.

In India, it has been our experience as clinical care providers that families are deeply involved in making decisions about a loved one's care, even in palliative and end-of-life scenarios [6]. Sparsh Hospice embraces this cultural reality by treating the patient and family as a single unit. While family involvement is encouraged and respected, the autonomy of the patient remains paramount. Upholding patient autonomy and advocating for their preferences are central to Sparsh Hospice's philosophy. This ensures that decisions about care, whether they pertain to active palliative support or hospice care, are guided by the patient's wishes while involving the family in a meaningful way. This is consistent with other global practices and priorities in palliative care to address what might otherwise be viewed as unmet need, which is not just about the patient, but the caring environment.

The referral system at Sparsh Hospice is also uniquely inclusive. Unlike traditional systems where referrals primarily come from treating hospitals, Sparsh Hospice receives patients through various channels, including social media, word of mouth, and recommendations from former beneficiaries. This broad referral base reflects the trust and reputation Sparsh Hospice has built in the community. Despite these diverse referral sources, admissions are handled with the utmost care. Every case undergoes a thorough evaluation by the in-house clinical team, ensuring that patients meet the criteria for palliative or hospice care. This process balances compassion with medical ethics, demonstrating a steadfast commitment to providing appropriate care without compromising on patient safety or intentions.

Sparsh Hospice's approach reflects a deep understanding of the complexities of palliative care in India. By expanding its scope, it has not only challenged the societal stigma surrounding palliative and hospice care but also reinforced the idea that these services are essential for anyone whose quality of life is severely impacted by illness. The organisation's work stands as a testament to its belief in patient autonomy, family-centric care, and holistic support systems that serve the needs of both patients and their loved ones.

3. Delivery framework: A humanistic bio-psycho-social model of compassionate, no-cost palliative care

At Sparsh Hospice, the care delivery framework is meticulously designed to address the diverse and complex needs of patients and their families, ensuring that palliative and hospice care is accessible, holistic, and compassionate. The organisation operates on a *biopsychosocial model of care*, recognising the interconnectedness of physical, emotional, social, and spiritual dimensions of a patient's well-being. This model acknowledges the unique cultural context of India, where families play an integral role in medical decision-making and caregiving, ensuring that both patients and their families are treated as a cohesive unit.

The care at Sparsh Hospice is delivered through three primary models:

3.1 Inpatient facility

Sparsh Hospice operates a state-of-the-art *82-bedded inpatient facility*, where patients are admitted for comprehensive palliative care and hospice care. This facility provides tailored care for patients in various stages of illness:

- *Palliative care admissions* are for individuals requiring intensive symptom management and relief from physical and emotional suffering.
- *Hospice care admissions* are designed for terminally ill patients, focusing on dignity, comfort, and quality of life during their final stages.
- *Respite care admissions* offer short-term stays to provide relief for families and caregivers who may be experiencing burnout. This ensures that both patients and their caregivers receive the support they need, maintaining the continuity of compassionate care.

3.2 Home care services

For patients unable to travel or access inpatient care, Sparsh Hospice provides *extensive home care services* within a 100-kilometre radius of Hyderabad. This model allows patients to receive comprehensive care in the comfort of their homes. A dedicated team, consisting of a physician, nurse, nursing aide (or bed-bound care assistant), and social counsellor, visits patients periodically to:

- Assess their medical and emotional needs.
- Provide symptom management and medications.
- Offer counselling, both emotional and spiritual, to patients and their families.

This personalised approach ensures continuity of care while respecting the patient's preference to remain in a familiar environment.

3.3 Outpatient services

For patients residing beyond the reach of the home care radius or those who prefer to visit the facility, Sparsh Hospice offers *outpatient services*. These services include:

DOI: http://dx.doi.org/10.5772/intechopen.1009161

- Consultations with physicians for palliative care planning and management.
- Necessary nursing procedures.
- Distribution of medications and personal care supplies.
- Counselling sessions to address emotional, social, or spiritual concerns.

Patients and their families can periodically walk into the facility, access the services they need, and return home with the required resources, ensuring uninterrupted care.

3.4 Expanding access to care

Sparsh Hospice [7] has made significant strides in ensuring that access to palliative care is not limited by geographical boundaries. While home care services are provided throughout Hyderabad, the organisation serves patients from across India, and occasionally, even international patients have availed themselves of its compassionate care. The organisation's philosophy of operating largely outside reimbursement [8] facilities ensures that care is prioritised based on need rather than financial constraints, allowing it to reach a wider demographic.

3.5 Delivery framework

The delivery framework at Sparsh Hospice is grounded in the *biopsychosocial model of care*, which acknowledges that the experience of illness extends beyond physical symptoms. This model integrates physical, psychological, social, and spiritual care to address the multifaceted suffering experienced by patients and their families.

In the Indian context, where families are deeply involved in medical decisions, this framework ensures that care is family-centric while upholding the patient's autonomy. Families are engaged in discussions and decisions, ensuring they feel supported while respecting the patient's wishes. The interdisciplinary team—comprising physicians, nurses, counsellors, and social workers—collaborates to provide care that is not just patient-focused but also family-inclusive.

By addressing the full spectrum of needs and recognising the cultural nuances of caregiving in India, Sparsh Hospice's care models and delivery framework set a benchmark for holistic, patient-centred, and family-centric palliative care.

3.6 Commitment to holistic care

Sparsh Hospice's care models and delivery framework are deeply rooted in its vision of providing holistic, patient-centred care. Whether through inpatient services, home care programs, or outpatient facilities, every aspect of its operations is designed to uphold the dignity and autonomy of patients while recognising the critical role of families in the care process. This holistic approach, supported by a multidisciplinary team and a robust operational structure, ensures that Sparsh Hospice continues to set a benchmark in palliative care.

4. Secular and inclusive care

In India, a nation celebrated for its multi-religious and secular fabric, palliative and hospice care must uphold these values to provide truly inclusive [9] and compassionate services. At Sparsh Hospice, the personal beliefs, cultural practices, and religious sentiments of patients and their families are deeply respected and seamlessly integrated into the care provided. This approach ensures that every patient experiences care that aligns with their individual values, fostering a sense of dignity and emotional well-being.

4.1 Celebrating diversity and preserving normalcy

To honour the diverse cultural and religious backgrounds of its patients, Sparsh Hospice adopts a secular approach to caregiving. Festivals from all religions are celebrated with enthusiasm, creating an environment of inclusivity and joy. Special occasions such as *birthdays* and *wedding anniversaries* of patients and their families are also celebrated, helping preserve a sense of normalcy in their lives despite the challenges posed by illness. These moments of joy and togetherness are carefully designed to remind patients that their identities and cherished milestones remain unaltered by their disease.

By facilitating such celebrations, Sparsh Hospice not only enhances the emotional and psychological well-being of its patients but also strengthens the bond between patients, families, and the caregiving team. This effort reinforces the organisation's commitment to providing holistic care that goes beyond physical relief to encompass emotional and spiritual fulfilment.

4.2 Navigating complex family dynamics

In India, families often comprise members with different religious beliefs coexisting harmoniously. This reality adds a unique dimension to caregiving, requiring sensitivity and adaptability from the care team. Sparsh Hospice recognises this complexity and trains its multidisciplinary team to handle such delicate dynamics with empathy and professionalism. Care is tailored to ensure that the diverse needs of each family are met without compromising the beliefs or comfort of any member.

4.3 Empowering the team for secular care

To provide care in a truly secular and inclusive manner, the Sparsh Hospice team is equipped with the knowledge and skills needed to respect and accommodate diverse belief systems. Regular training sessions are conducted to sensitise the staff to the cultural and religious practices of different communities. This ensures that all interactions with patients and families are conducted with the utmost respect and understanding.

4.4 Upholding emotional well-being

Sparsh Hospice understands that illness can profoundly impact a patient's sense of identity and emotional well-being. By respecting their beliefs, celebrating milestones, and fostering a secular and inclusive environment, the organisation works to preserve the emotional resilience of patients and families. This care philosophy ensures that patients feel valued and supported, allowing them to experience peace and comfort throughout their journey. Specific steps are taken to get feedback from patients and families about the care received.

5. Enhancing quality of life

At Sparsh Hospice, enhancing the quality of life for patients goes beyond addressing their physical symptoms. The organisation understands that the *quality of life* is deeply personal and varies from one individual to another. For some, it may mean regaining a sense of autonomy; for others, it could be fulfilling small desires, enjoying moments of joy with loved ones, or even reliving cherished experiences. Sparsh Hospice strives to create these meaningful moments, tailoring its approach to each patient's unique preferences and aspirations.

5.1 Fulfilling individual needs

Recognising that the quality of life is multifaceted, Sparsh Hospice facilitates a variety of activities and experiences for its patients, including:

- *Outings and excursions*: Organising car rides, visits to nearby temples, or even trips to the cinema to ensure patients experience moments of joy and connection with the outside world.

- *Family visits*: Creating opportunities for patients to spend meaningful time with their families in the inpatient facility, fostering a sense of belonging and emotional support.

Additionally, Sparsh Hospice goes the extra mile to fulfil patients' specific wishes, whether it is arranging for a favourite cricket star or movie star to visit them or helping them experience a long-held dream. These efforts demonstrate the organisation's commitment to treating patients as individuals and honouring their unique desires.

5.2 Creating a positive ambience

A significant aspect of enhancing the quality of life at Sparsh Hospice lies in the creation of an *uplifting and positive environment*. The inpatient facility is designed to ensure patients feel comforted and valued, rather than overwhelmed by the weight of their illness. This is achieved through a variety of initiatives:

- *Cultural activities*: Events featuring artists, singers, dancers, and performers are organised regularly, bringing joy and entertainment to the patients.

- *Art workshops*: Patients can participate in creative activities, allowing them to express themselves and engage their minds in meaningful ways.

- *Engagement with the community*: Visits from school children and community groups create an atmosphere of vitality and connection, reminding patients that they are an integral part of society.

- *The library*: Patients have access to a library where a diverse collection of books, including secular literature and other genres, ensures there is something for everyone.

- *The garden*: Provides a serene outdoor space where visitors can relax and enjoy a peaceful ambience.
- *The amphitheatre*: An amphitheatre where patients gather not only to enjoy cultural activities but also to socialise with families and fellow caregivers during gatherings.

These initiatives are curated to help patients focus on the present moment, fostering positivity even as they face the challenges of illness.

5.3 Preserving normalcy in home care

The commitment to preserving normalcy and enhancing quality of life extends beyond the walls of Sparsh Hospice's inpatient facility. In its *home care services*, the team makes special efforts to celebrate important milestones and festivals with patients and their families in the comfort of their homes.

- *Facilitate the celebration of festivals* at home with warmth and reflection, ensuring they align with the cultural and religious traditions of the patient and their family.
- *Community lunches* are organised, fostering a sense of togetherness and shared joy for patients, caregivers, and their communities.
- *Birthdays, wedding anniversaries, and other special days* are acknowledged and celebrated, creating opportunities for joy and connection amidst challenging circumstances.

By incorporating these practices into its home care programs, Sparsh Hospice ensures that the emotional and social well-being of patients and families is prioritised, regardless of location.

5.4 Preserving normalcy

Sparsh Hospice recognises the importance of *preserving a sense of normalcy* in the lives of its patients. Illness may alter physical capabilities, but it should not diminish their ability to experience joy, fulfil desires, or participate in life's meaningful moments. The team works tirelessly to ensure that patients feel supported, loved, and valued, giving them a sense of purpose and dignity.

By creating a space where patients can celebrate life through personalised care, cultural engagement, and cherished experiences, Sparsh Hospice truly redefines the concept of quality of life in the context of palliative care.

6. Resource and equipment accessibility

At Sparsh Hospice, enhancing the quality of life is not limited to providing medical care but extends to offering a range of support services that address the holistic needs of patients and their families. By facilitating access to essential equipment,

DOI: http://dx.doi.org/10.5772/intechopen.1009161

seasonal and nutritional support, and social resources, Sparsh Hospice ensures that both patients and caregivers experience a sense of physical and emotional comfort throughout the caregiving journey.

6.1 Equipment support for home care patients

Sparsh Hospice recognises the unique challenges faced by families caring for patients at home. To alleviate the financial and logistical burdens associated with home-based care, the organisation provides access to a variety of essential medical equipment and supplies, including:

- *Oxygen support* such as concentrators, ensuring patients have uninterrupted respiratory care.
- *Medical cots and airbeds* to enhance patient comfort and prevent complications such as bedsores.
- *Suction machines and nebulisers* to manage respiratory issues effectively.
- *Commode chairs, walkers, and mobility aids*, enabling patients to maintain some degree of independence and dignity.

These resources are shared with families as part of Sparsh Hospice's commitment to reducing the strain on caregivers and creating a more comfortable and dignified environment for patients. By making such equipment readily accessible, Sparsh Hospice not only provides physical relief to patients but also offers emotional reassurance to families, knowing that their loved ones are receiving the best possible care at home.

6.2 Comprehensive support for inpatient and home care patients

At its *inpatient facility*, Sparsh Hospice provides a wide range of services free of cost, including:

- *Medications* to manage symptoms and improve quality of life.
- *Nutritional support*, offering specialised dietary plans tailored to each patient's needs.
- *Round-the-clock medical care* provided by physicians, nurses, and other healthcare professionals.
- *Comfortable accommodations* that ensure a positive and healing environment for patients and families.

For patients in the *home care program*, Sparsh Hospice extends similar support by coordinating the provision of essential resources. In addition to medical equipment, the team facilitates the delivery of *seasonal necessities* such as blankets during winter and other items required to enhance patient comfort.

6.3 Addressing nutritional and social needs

Sparsh Hospice goes beyond medical care to provide *nutritional and social support* to families in need, recognising the financial and emotional strain that serious illness often places on households. For families where the primary breadwinner is the patient, Sparsh Hospice works through its extensive network to supply:

- *Dry groceries*, ensuring that the family's basic needs are met.
- *Nutritional supplements*, tailored to the requirements of patients with specific dietary needs.

7. Spiritual and psychological support

In palliative and hospice care, addressing the spiritual and psychological needs of patients is indispensable for providing holistic care. At Sparsh Hospice, these aspects are carefully evaluated and addressed, recognising that the journey of illness affects not only the body but also the mind and spirit.

7.1 Spiritual support

In a multi-religious and secular society like India, Sparsh Hospice acknowledges the diverse belief systems of its patients and families. The team is trained to respect and accommodate religious beliefs, even if they fall outside the purview of their personal experiences or understanding. This inclusivity fosters an environment of mutual respect and ensures that spiritual needs are met with sincerity and care.

The spiritual needs of patients are assessed periodically, and efforts are made to fulfil their specific requests, which may include:

- Organising religious functions or rituals at the facility.
- Arranging visits to nearby places of worship.
- Facilitating prayers or spiritual gatherings for the patient and their family.

7.2 Psychological support

The emotional state of patients evolves as their illness progresses, and Sparsh Hospice places a strong emphasis on providing psychological support to help patients and families navigate these changes. A dedicated team of counsellors, psychologists, and social workers works closely with patients and families to:

- Conduct *individual counselling sessions* for patients to address their fears, anxieties, and changing emotions.
- Facilitate *family counselling sessions* to help families adapt to the evolving dynamics of care and strengthen their ability to support the patient.
- Hold *caregiver meetings* to address caregiver burnout, ensure effective communication, and resolve any conflicts that may arise within the family.

7.3 Ensuring harmony and facilitating a good death

Sparsh Hospice understands that family dynamics can be complex and fluid during a patient's illness. To address these challenges, the organisation fosters open communication and collaboration among family members to ensure that patient care remains uninterrupted. By providing a safe space for families to share concerns and seek guidance, Sparsh Hospice helps create a harmonious environment that supports the patient's journey.

The ultimate goal of this comprehensive approach is to facilitate a *good death*—a peaceful and dignified transition for the patient, free from unnecessary suffering. This is achieved by aligning care with the patient's spiritual and emotional needs while supporting the family through their own journey of acceptance and adjustment.

8. Mortuary and end-of-life services

Sparsh Hospice extends its compassionate care beyond the patient's life by offering *free mortuary and end-of-life services*, ensuring that families are supported during one of the most difficult times. These services are designed to accommodate the unique needs of families, including those who may be geographically dispersed or facing financial constraints.

8.1 Free mortuary services

Recognising the challenges families face when they are spread across different locations, Sparsh Hospice provides a *free mortuary facility* where the mortal remains of patients can be respectfully preserved for up to a week. This service allows families the time needed to gather and pay their respects without added financial burden. By facilitating this service with care and dignity, Sparsh Hospice ensures that families can focus on mourning and honouring their loved ones without undue stress.

8.2 Funeral services

In partnership with nearby funeral service providers, Sparsh Hospice also offers *free funeral services* for families who may not have the financial resources to organise them. This includes coordinating the necessary arrangements to ensure a dignified farewell for the patient, aligned with the family's cultural and religious practices. These services are a vital part of Sparsh Hospice's commitment to holistic care, extending its compassion to the very end of the patient's journey.

8.3 Respecting living wills and POLST orders

Sparsh Hospice upholds the autonomy of its patients by respecting *living wills* and *Physician Orders for Life-Sustaining Treatment (POLST) documents*. These directives guide the care provided during the patient's final stages and ensure that their end-of-life preferences are honoured. The organisation works closely with families to ensure these wishes are understood and followed, reinforcing its dedication to preserving the dignity and choices of every individual.

By providing free mortuary services, facilitating funerals for those in need, and respecting end-of-life directives, Sparsh Hospice demonstrates its unwavering commitment to compassionate and inclusive care. These services are an integral part of its philosophy of ensuring dignity and respect, even in death.

9. Bereavement support

Sparsh Hospice extends its care and compassion beyond the passing of a patient by offering comprehensive *bereavement support* to families. Recognising the deep rapport formed with families during the care journey, the team often participates in funeral services or post-funeral rituals as per the wishes of the patient or the family's belief system. This involvement reflects Sparsh Hospice's commitment to being a part of the family's healing process, respecting their traditions, and offering emotional comfort during a challenging time.

9.1 Memorial services

Sparsh Hospice facilitates *memorial lunches or dinners*, providing families with a space to honour their loved ones while fostering a sense of closure and community. These services, hosted at the facility, serve as an opportunity for families to come together, share memories, and find solace in a supportive environment.

9.2 Long-term bereavement support

Understanding that grief is a prolonged process, Sparsh Hospice provides *15 months of follow-up bereavement support* to families. During this period, the team maintains periodic contact to

- Address emotional concerns and offer counselling when needed.
- Provide referrals or resources for additional support.

9.3 Networking for livelihoods and education

To further assist families during this transitional phase, Sparsh Hospice networks with other organisations to help secure *alternative livelihoods* for families who may have lost their primary breadwinner. Additionally, connections are facilitated for *children's education programs*, ensuring that families can rebuild their lives with stability and support.

10. Fostering team welfare and professional excellence

At Sparsh Hospice, the well-being, growth, and recognition of the staff are considered essential for delivering compassionate and high-quality palliative care. Investing in continuous professional development, ensuring a supportive work environment, and prioritising the health of the team is integral to maintaining the highest standards of care for patients and their families.

10.1 Continuum of education and professional growth

Sparsh Hospice is committed to fostering the continuous professional development of its staff, enabling them to stay at the forefront of advancements in palliative care. Key initiatives include:

- *Education support*: Staff are encouraged to pursue higher qualifications, certifications, and specialised training in palliative care and related fields, with financial assistance provided to reduce the burden of these pursuits.

- *Skill development*: Regular in-house training sessions, workshops, and educational programs are organised to enhance both technical expertise and interpersonal skills. A state-of-the-art audio-visual room is available, thoughtfully designed to support training programs and workshops, ensuring an engaging and impactful learning environment.

- *Access to literature*: A library with a comprehensive collection of palliative care literature is made accessible to staff, allowing them to upscale their knowledge and stay informed about the latest practices.

- *Global exposure*: Participation in international conferences, workshops, and forums is facilitated, providing staff with insights into global best practices and innovative approaches in palliative care.

- *Knowledge contributions*: Staff are supported in presenting research papers, participating in poster sessions, and contributing to collaborative projects, fostering professional growth while advancing the field of palliative care.

By prioritising education and skill enhancement, Sparsh Hospice ensures that staff members are equipped to provide care aligned with the latest standards while encouraging their professional growth.

10.2 Staff well-being and team support

Recognising the physical and emotional demands of palliative care, Sparsh Hospice takes active measures to support the health, well-being, and morale of its staff. Initiatives include:

- *Vaccination programs*: Necessary vaccinations are prioritised for the staff, including Hepatitis B, HPV (cervical cancer), and COVID-19 vaccines, ensuring their health and safety.

- *Ongoing medical support*: Staff members are provided with free access to ongoing medical support, including medications for themselves and their families from the organisation's pharmacy, at no additional cost.

- *Subsidised meals*: Nutritious food is made available at subsidised rates for staff on regular working days.

- *Well-being sessions*: Periodic mental health and resilience workshops are conducted to promote emotional well-being.
- *Debriefing sessions*: Safe spaces are provided for staff to share their experiences, reflect on challenges, and receive emotional support.
- *Recreational and relaxation activities*: Yoga sessions, team-building exercises, and leisure programs are organised to foster camaraderie and relaxation.
- *Celebrating festivals and milestones*: Gala dinners, festival-specific lunches, and celebrations of achievements are held regularly to foster a sense of community and recognition.
- *Gifting and recognition*: Periodic gifting of clothes and other thoughtful tokens of appreciation is carried out to acknowledge the dedication of staff members.

These initiatives are designed to create a supportive, nurturing, and health-conscious work environment where staff feel valued, motivated, and equipped to provide the best possible care.

11. Community awareness and engagement

Sparsh Hospice recognises that the barriers to palliative care—such as societal stigma, lack of awareness, and limited accessibility—must be addressed proactively to ensure broader acceptance and reach. To achieve this, the organisation conducts extensive *awareness programs* across multiple levels, involving various communities and stakeholders. These initiatives aim to remove taboos surrounding palliative care and foster a culture of compassion and understanding.

11.1 Multi-level awareness programs

Awareness programs are conducted both within the city of Hyderabad and in the rural areas of Telangana. These programs are carried out in collaboration with:

- *Government health systems*, including primary health care centres and ground-level health care workers, to ensure the message reaches underserved populations.
- *Corporate offices*, creating awareness among employees and fostering a sense of social responsibility.
- *Residential communities*, encouraging individuals to understand the importance of palliative care and how they can contribute to its acceptance.
- *Schools and educational institutions*, where sessions are conducted to nurture empathy and compassion in younger generations.

These efforts are designed to not only increase accessibility to palliative care but also encourage communities to embrace its significance in improving the quality of life for patients and their families.

DOI: http://dx.doi.org/10.5772/intechopen.1009161

11.2 Integrating palliative care into education

As part of its commitment to creating *compassionate communities*, Sparsh Hospice has successfully integrated palliative care concepts into the *IB curriculum (International Baccalaureate)* under the Creativity, Activity, Service (CAS) program. This initiative helps schoolchildren understand the importance of palliative care, fostering empathy and teaching them how to support individuals living with illnesses or facing crises. Through this program, Sparsh Hospice aims to build a future generation that is compassionate, informed, and prepared to address the challenges of caregiving with sensitivity and care.

12. Advocacy for end-of-life choices and legal awareness

Sparsh Hospice has been at the forefront of advocating for informed end-of-life care decisions, fostering awareness among patients and families about their rights, and encouraging dignity in care during the final stages of life. With its recent empanelment under the *Rajiv Aarogyasri* [1], *Telangana state* [2] the organisation has intensified its efforts to make palliative and hospice care more accessible and accepted, while simultaneously addressing the evolving legal and ethical dimensions of end-of-life care.

12.1 Encouraging living wills and proxy decision makers

A key focus of Sparsh Hospice's advocacy is empowering patients to take an active role in planning their care. The organisation encourages individuals to consider creating *living wills* or appoint *proxy healthcare decision makers* to ensure that their preferences for end-of-life care are respected. By initiating conversations about these choices, Sparsh Hospice helps patients and families:

- Understand the importance of having clear directives for medical interventions.
- Ensure that care decisions align with their values and beliefs.
- Foster open communication within families to reduce conflicts during critical moments.

12.2 Promoting awareness of legal provisions

Since 2023, significant legal advancements in India have allowed for the *withholding and withdrawal of futile medical interventions* under certain circumstances. Sparsh Hospice has taken a proactive approach to raising awareness about these provisions, ensuring that patients and families understand the legal framework and its implications. During counselling sessions and community engagements, the team:

- Educates families about the options available under current laws.
- Explains scenarios where these decisions can be made to uphold the dignity and comfort of the patient.
- Provides guidance on how to document and formalise these choices, ensuring compliance with legal standards.

Sparsh Hospice firmly believes in the concept of *dignity in end-of-life care*, advocating for care that prioritises comfort, respect, and autonomy. By addressing topics like living wills, advanced medical directives, and legal permissions, the organisation helps families and patients make informed choices that reflect their wishes and ensure a peaceful transition.

13. Economic sustainability

The ability to offer palliative and hospice care free of cost to patients with serious health-related issues requires a robust framework of economic sustainability. Sparsh Hospice, managed by the *Rotary Club of Banjara Hills Charitable Trust*, has successfully built a strong foundation of financial support through its goodwill, partnerships, and community impact.

Sparsh Hospice demonstrates its commitment to sustainability by using recycled water for gardening, harnessing solar energy, and adopting rainwater harvesting practices, effectively balancing environmental care with cost efficiency.

13.1 Support through CSR and philanthropy

The organisation's commitment to providing care without financial barriers has garnered widespread support from various stakeholders, including:

- *Corporate Social Responsibility (CSR)* [3] *contributions* from prominent companies, which recognise the value of Sparsh Hospice's work in improving community well-being.

- *Government support*, particularly through programs like the Rajiv Aarogyasri (Telangana- state) Government Healthcare Insurance Scheme, further bolsters the sustainability of its services.

- *Individual philanthropists* who are deeply moved by the cause and contribute generously to ensure the continuity of care.

These partnerships not only help sustain the day-to-day operations of the hospice but also enable it to expand its services, ensuring that no patient is turned away due to financial constraints.

13.2 Adding value to the community

Sparsh Hospice's model of care does more than address physical suffering; it fosters a sense of dignity and emotional well-being for patients during their end-of-life journey. The organisation's impact extends to families and communities, who find comfort in knowing that their loved ones receive compassionate, holistic care without financial burden. This approach eliminates any sense of self-pity, replacing it with a profound sense of respect and acceptance, both for the patient and their families.

By combining compassionate care with strong economic sustainability, Sparsh Hospice serves as a beacon of hope and goodwill, ensuring that the invaluable service of palliative and hospice care continues to uplift countless lives.

14. The role of volunteers

Volunteers are a vital part of the care ecosystem at Sparsh Hospice, contributing significantly to raising awareness, mobilising resources, and creating a network of support for patients and families. Their efforts enhance the reach and impact of palliative care within communities.

14.1 Awareness and resource mobilisation

Volunteers play a key role in spreading awareness about palliative care, and participating in community engagement activities to educate and encourage early intervention. They also help mobilise in-kind donations, such as medical supplies, clothing, and other essentials, ensuring that patients' needs are met. Additionally, their efforts in connecting with donors and sponsors sustain the operational and financial stability of the hospice.

14.2 Referrals and community support

Through their community networks, volunteers identify and refer patients to Sparsh Hospice, facilitating access to timely care. They also contribute to building a support system for patients and their families, offering emotional and social assistance during challenging times.

14.3 Structured volunteer program

In collaboration with the Indian Association of Palliative Care (IAPC), Sparsh Hospice conducts a structured community volunteer training program. This initiative equips volunteers with the knowledge and skills required to provide effective support while encouraging long-term community volunteer behaviour.

15. Conclusion

Sparsh Hospice stands as a testament to the power of compassion, inclusivity, and community-driven care. Over the years, the organisation has successfully redefined palliative and hospice care in India, creating a model that is patient-centric, holistic, and deeply empathetic. By addressing not only the physical suffering of patients but also their emotional, social, and spiritual needs, Sparsh Hospice has set a benchmark for end-of-life care that upholds dignity and enhances quality of life.

Through its unwavering commitment to accessibility and inclusivity, Sparsh Hospice has been able to serve over *11,500 beneficiaries* directly, while supporting countless families as *indirect beneficiaries*. This impact extends beyond the patients themselves, touching the lives of caregivers, families, and communities by fostering a culture of acceptance, compassion, and understanding.

The ability to provide care free of cost is supported by CSR funding [10], government collaborations, and philanthropic contributions, highlighting the strength of its economic sustainability model. The National Corporate Social Responsibility (CSR) is a commitment by businesses that contribute to the social and environmental well-being of the communities in which they operate. CSR can take many forms, including philanthropy, volunteering, and environmental initiatives. One way that businesses can support CSR is by providing funding to NGOs. NGOs are non-profit organisations that work to address social and environmental issues. By providing funding to NGOs, businesses can help to make a real difference in the world.

With CSR support Sparsh is able to focus on integrating advocacy, education, and community engagement into its operations. The care setting has also succeeded in challenging societal taboos, increasing awareness, and creating pathways for future acceptance and accessibility of palliative care.

As Sparsh Hospice continues to grow, its mission remains steadfast: to ensure that no patient faces their journey alone and that every individual receives the care, respect, and dignity they deserve. This legacy of compassion not only uplifts the patients and their families but also enriches the community, building a more humane and empathetic society for generations to come. Furthermore, palliative care which comes from the West, has unique challenges in India's healthcare system. The important conclusions of this chapter are to emphasise that providing palliative care outside regular healthcare payment methods, especially in non-profit healthcare, is beneficial. It focuses on giving patients more control, caring for their specific needs, and being flexible with who can get help, even if they are expected to live longer than six months [11].

Author details

Padma Sesha Sarada Lingaraju
Sparsh Hospice, Hyderabad, India

*Address all correspondence to: hospadministrator@sparshhospice.org

References

[1] Aarogyasri Health Care Trust. Ministry of Corporate Affairs Government of Inida. Beneficiaries Covered and Financial Coverage Provided; n.d. Available from: https://health.vikaspedia.in/viewcontent/health/nrhm/state-health-programmes/aarogyasri-of-telangana?lgn=en [Accessed: January 12, 2024]

[2] Telangana State: Health, Medical and Family Welfare. Available from: www.telangana.gov.in/departments/health-medical-family-welfare [Accessed: January 12, 2024]

[3] Flieger SP, Chui K, Koch-Weser S. Lack of awareness and common misconceptions about palliative care among adults: Insights from a national survey. Journal of General Internal Medicine. 2020;**35**(7):2059-2064. DOI: 10.1007/s11606-020-05730-4

[4] World Health Organization. WHO Definition of Palliative Care. Geneva: WHO; 2021. Available from: https://www.who.int/cancer/palliative/definition/en/

[5] Meier DE, Back AL, Berman A, Block SD, Corrigan JM, Morrison RS. A national strategy for palliative care. Health Affairs. 2017;**36**(7):1265-1273. DOI: 10.1377/hlthaff.2017.0164

[6] Shukla R, Singh N, Acharya S, Shukla S. Hospice care in India: A review. Journal of Family Medicine and Primary Care. 2022;**11**(9):4987-4990. DOI: 10.4103/jfmpc.jfmpc_2265_21

[7] Global Directory of Palliative Care Institutions and Organizations-International Association for Hospice and Palliative. IAHPC Annual Report; 2021. Available from: https://hospicecare.com/global-directory-of-providers-organizations/search/?idcountry=39 [Accessed: December 10, 2024]

[8] Lingaraju PSS. Advantages of palliative care outside healthcare financing schemes in nonprofit healthcare settings in the Indian context recognition of suffering prior to last six months. Journal of Palliative Care and Medicine. 2024;**14**(3):624-626

[9] Barrett NJ, Bullock K, Johnson KS. Unmet needs in health disparities research—It's not just about patients. JAMA Internal Medicine. 2022;**182**(9):995-996. DOI: 10.1001/jamainternmed.2022.2877

[10] Jones T, Nedjat-Haiem F, Bullock K. Health equity in palliative care. In: Altilio T, Otis-Green S, editors. Oxford Textbook of Palliative Social Work. New York, NY: Oxford University Press; 2022. pp. 14-25

[11] National Corporate Social Responsibility. Report of the High Level Committee; n.d. Available from: https://csr.gov.in/ [Accessed: January 12, 2024]

Chapter 12

Cultural Acceptance of Palliative Care in Arab Societies

Amna Al-Harrasi, Nasr Al-Riyami, Atika AlMusalami, Rawan AlMujaini, Entesar AlYafai, Nawal Al Mahyijari and Adhari Al Zaabi

Abstract

This chapter examines the cultural acceptance of palliative care in Arab societies, emphasizing the interplay between historical, religious, and cultural factors that shape perceptions and practices around end-of-life care. Palliative care remains underdeveloped in many Arab countries due to stigma, limited awareness, and systemic challenges such as restricted access to opioids and inadequate professional training. Islamic teachings, family-centered care traditions, and societal norms significantly influence healthcare decision-making, often balancing spiritual preparation for death with patient care needs. Psychosocial complexities, including the emotional and mental burdens on patients and families, further highlight the necessity of culturally sensitive communication and holistic care approaches. While countries like Jordan and Saudi Arabia have made progress in integrating palliative care, significant disparities persist, particularly in rural and underserved areas. Addressing these challenges requires fostering cultural acceptance through community engagement, education campaigns, and the involvement of religious leaders. Additionally, future efforts must prioritize national policies, capacity building, and research tailored to local contexts to ensure equitable access to palliative care services. By recognizing and respecting cultural and religious values, healthcare systems can better meet the needs of terminally ill patients and their families, ultimately improving quality of life and care outcomes.

Keywords: palliative care, Arab societies, cultural acceptance, end-of-life care, Islamic teachings, Muslims, Arabs

1. Introduction

1.1 Definition of palliative care

Palliative care is defined by the *World Health Organization (WHO)* as *"the specialized medical care for people living with a serious, complex, or terminal illness. It focuses on providing relief from pain and other distressing symptoms and addressing psychological, social, and spiritual concerns.*" Palliative care differs from curative treatments in that it prioritizes quality of life rather than solely focusing on disease eradication [1]. The *National Consensus Project for Quality Palliative Care* (NCP) further emphasizes its multidisciplinary approach, involving medical, emotional, psychological, and spiritual care for patients and their families [2]. Palliative care can be provided alongside curative treatments or as the main focus of care when curative treatments are no longer effective.

1.2 Importance of cultural context in healthcare

Cultural context shapes healthcare practices, attitudes, and illness and treatment perceptions. Beliefs, traditions, religious values, and social norms influence the acceptance and delivery of medical interventions. For instance, cultural attitudes toward death, dying, and care at the end of life can significantly determine how palliative care is understood and implemented [3]. In Arab societies, cultural and religious values intersect, creating unique challenges and opportunities for palliative care acceptance and integration into healthcare services. Understanding these dynamics is essential for fostering trust and ensuring that care is sensitive, respectful, and responsive to individual and communal needs [4].

1.3 Overview of psychosocial oncology and its relevance to palliative care

Psychosocial oncology addresses the emotional, social, and psychological needs of patients with cancer and their families throughout the trajectory of illness. It integrates mental health care into the broader scope of oncology treatment, recognizing that emotional and psychological well-being is integral to patients' quality of life [5]. Within palliative care, psychosocial oncology serves as a bridge between physical symptom management and addressing mental health concerns, such as depression, anxiety, or grief. The inclusion of psychosocial interventions can alleviate the emotional suffering often experienced by individuals facing end-of-life issues [6]. Effective psychosocial care requires cultural sensitivity and an understanding of how different cultural groups conceptualize illness, suffering, and coping mechanisms.

1.4 Objectives of the chapter

Arab countries, also known as the Arab world, refer to a group of 22 countries that are members of the Arab League. These countries share a common cultural and linguistic heritage, with Arabic being the predominant language. The Arab world spans two continents: Asia and Africa.

The primary objective of this chapter is to explore the cultural acceptance of palliative care within Arab societies, highlighting the intricate interplay between cultural beliefs, religious values, and psychosocial factors that influence end-of-life care. We aim to comprehensively understand how these cultural dimensions shape perceptions of palliative care, including its accessibility and integration into healthcare systems. Additionally, the chapter seeks to identify the psychosocial complexities patients and families face, emphasizing the need for culturally sensitive approaches in care practices.

By examining current challenges and barriers, such as stigma, lack of awareness, and differing attitudes toward death and dying, this chapter aspires to propose actionable strategies for enhancing the acceptance and implementation of palliative care. These strategies aim to foster culturally appropriate interventions and education campaigns, strengthen support networks, and address gaps in access to healthcare services. Ultimately, the goal is to improve the quality of life for patients and their families by ensuring that palliative care is responsive to the cultural and religious values of Arab communities.

2. Cultural context of palliative care in the Arab world

2.1 Historical perspectives on end-of-life care

In Arab societies, the approach to end-of-life care has deep historical and cultural roots shaped by pre-Islamic traditions, the rise of Islam, and advancements during the medieval Islamic Golden Age (**Figure 1**).

2.1.1 Pre-Islamic era

Before the advent of Islam, Arab tribes had diverse customs and traditions around death and dying. These practices varied widely among tribes but generally included ritualistic mourning and strong community support for grieving families. Death was seen as a natural part of life, and care for the dying was primarily communal, with the extended family and tribal structures offering emotional and practical support during illness and death [7].

2.1.2 Islamic influence

With the advent of Islam in the seventh century, Islamic teachings began to shape end-of-life care practices profoundly. Islamic principles emphasize the sanctity of life, the inevitability of death, and the importance of preparing for the afterlife.

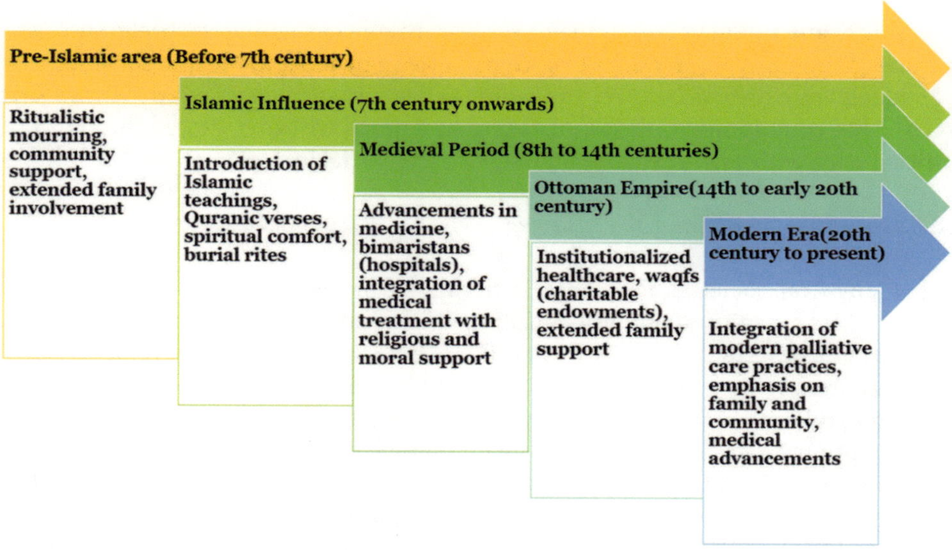

Figure 1.
Historical perspective on end-of-life care in Arab societies.

Practices such as reciting Quranic verses, such as reciting Surah Yasin (a chapter from the Quran) to the ill and dying and offering du'a (prayers), provide spiritual comfort for both patients and their families [8]. The prophet Mohammed's teaching included remedies and medicines that, in the majority, targeted symptom management rather than cure.

2.1.3 Medieval period

The Islamic Golden Age (8th to 14th centuries) brought significant advancements in healthcare. Scholars such as Ibn Sina (Avicenna) and Al-Razi integrated medical, ethical, and spiritual care into practice. Hospitals, known as baristas, were established to provide comprehensive care for the sick and dying. This era emphasized compassionate care, reflecting Islamic humanitarian values [9].

2.1.4 Ottoman empire

The Ottoman era was institutionalized through Waqfs (charitable endowments), which funded hospitals and care centers, ensuring free access to care for the poor and needy. Families remained the cornerstone of care provision, offering emotional and practical support alongside hospital services [10].

2.1.5 Modern era

In contemporary times, integrating modern palliative care practices with traditional and religious values has become more pronounced. Arab societies continue to emphasize the importance of family and community in end-of-life care while incorporating medical advancements and palliative care principles to improve patients' quality of life [11].

2.2 Cultural beliefs and values regarding death and dying

Cultural and religious beliefs play a significant role in shaping the preferences and attitudes of patients and families toward palliative care in Arab Muslim societies. For individuals from diverse cultural and religious backgrounds, particularly within Arab and Muslim communities, illness, suffering, and death are often viewed through a spiritual lens, with a firm reliance on religious and social interpretations [12, 13].

2.2.1 Attitudes toward illness and suffering

In many Arab societies, illness and suffering are perceived as tests of faith or opportunities for spiritual growth. Suffering is often seen as a way to attain spiritual rewards in the afterlife. This belief can influence care decisions, where patients may decline aggressive interventions in favor of spiritual preparation. However, it can also lead to reluctance to seek pain management or palliative interventions due to misconceptions that alleviating suffering might undermine faith [8, 14]. However, more recently in Arab cultures, many patients opt to remain hospitalized during their final days because hospitals are perceived as places of safety and specialized care. Motivated by love and cultural obligation, families often seek second opinions or additional interventions to "do everything possible" for loved ones, even when such measures involve aggressive medical interventions [12]. A prevalent misconception in

DOI: http://dx.doi.org/10.5772/intechopen.1009422

these contexts is the belief that opioids, such as morphine, cause addiction or hasten death, leading to widespread underutilization and poor pain management [13]. This misconception, combined with the stigma surrounding opioid use, hinders the effective delivery of palliative care services and exacerbates patients' suffering.

2.2.2 Family's role in care decisions

Arab culture emphasizes family collectivism, where care decisions are made collectively rather than individually. Families often prioritize protecting patients from distressing information about their prognosis, which may conflict with the concept of patient autonomy [15, 16]. While this approach ensures that patients are not left to face illness alone, it can hinder open communication and decision-making regarding end-of-life issues [12, 13].

2.3 Religious influences on palliative care practices

Islam provides a comprehensive framework for end care emphasizing compassion, dignity, and spiritual well-being.

2.3.1 Islamic teachings on end-of-life care

Islamic principles encourage the alleviation of suffering, with the use of pain relief (e.g., opioids) being permissible as long as it does not hasten death [17]. Prophecy Mohammed emphasized the importance of caring for the sick, reflecting humanitarian values. Practices such as Dhikr (remembrance of God) and salat (prayers) comfort dying patients.

2.3.2 Variations across different Arab cultures

While Islamic principles form a shared foundation, local traditions and interpretations of Islamic teachings introduce regional variation. For example, Gulf countries may emphasize stricter family involvement and religious practices compared to more diverse Levantine or North African societies. The extended family often assumes caregiving responsibilities at home, which is considered an act of spiritual and moral duty. Providing care in the house ensures privacy and allows families to uphold cultural values of honoring and supporting the patient in their final moments. These variations influence preferences for home-based care versus hospital care and attitudes toward aggressive interventions [18]. Furthermore, families may seek support from religious healers or traditional medicine practitioners alongside formal palliative care in rural or conventional parts of the Gulf and North Africa. Practices like Ruqyah (spiritual healing through Qur'anic verses) may accompany medical treatments [19, 20].

2.4 Palliative care terminology from the Quran and Arab cultural context

2.4.1 Quranic terminology and spiritual foundations

In Arab Muslim societies, palliative care draws heavily from Islamic principles rooted in the Quran and Hadith. The concept of rahma (mercy) is central to the care of those facing end-of-life challenges, as Allah is described as "The Most Merciful"

(Ar-Rahman) in the Quran. Another vital term is sabr (patience), frequently encouraged in the Quran during hardship and suffering. Patients and their families are often reminded of tawakkul (reliance on God), which signifies entrusting their circumstances to divine will, particularly when medical interventions can no longer cure illness. Such values provide spiritual comfort and align closely with the principles of palliative care, emphasizing compassion, dignity, and holistic support [7, 10, 15, 21].

2.4.2 Local terminologies in Arab societies

In the Arab world, cultural and linguistic nuances often shape palliative care-related terms. The term ri'aya takhfif al-alam (care to alleviate suffering) is widely used to describe palliative care, emphasizing the relief of pain and discomfort. Terms like ma'raka ma'al marad (battle with illness) reflect the cultural framing of illness as a challenge requiring endurance and faith. Additionally, the word yusr (ease) is significant, as it resonates with the Quranic verse, "Verily, with hardship comes ease" (Quran 94:6). This provides a spiritual framework for encouraging both patients and caregivers to find hope and peace amid struggles. Regional dialects might also employ phrases unique to specific communities, reflecting the interplay of traditional values with modern medical practices [7, 10, 15, 21].

In Oman, for example, we use "palliative care" translate to Arabic as "ar-ra'aya at-taltifiya"). This translation may be used in formal healthcare settings, documents, or discussions. The word "lutf or taltif" appears in several verses of the Quran. While it does not directly translate to "palliative care," it carries specific meanings that resonate with the principles and goals of palliative care, for example, kindness, gentleness, compassion, favor, grace, mercy, ease, comfort, and relief. Another terminology commonly used (ar-ri'ayah al-mukh hafifah li-l-a'rāḍ), which means "symptom-relieving care".

2.4.3 Integration of faith and care practices

Faith-based terminology in Arab countries bridges the gap between religious practices and palliative care interventions. For instance, concepts like ihsan (benevolence) and husn al-khatima (a good ending) align with the goals of ensuring a peaceful and dignified death. Religious leaders and chaplains often use these terms to counsel families and patients, facilitating acceptance of the terminal nature of illnesses while adhering to Islamic tenets. This integration ensures that the spiritual and emotional needs of the patients are met, alongside physical care. Moreover, using these terms by healthcare providers fosters culturally sensitive communication and trust, ensuring palliative care is more accessible and meaningful in Arab societies [7, 21].

These perspectives highlight the profound influence of Islamic teachings and local cultures on palliative care, encouraging holistic support grounded in faith, community, and compassion.

3. Current state of palliative care in Arab countries

Worldwide, around 40 million people need palliative care each year, with 78% of them living in low- and middle-income countries. This includes a significant number of non-cancer patients suffering from chronic illnesses such as heart disease, respiratory diseases, and neurological disorders. In the Eastern Mediterranean Region (EMRO), which includes many Arab countries, the need for palliative care is increasing [22]. For example, in Saudi Arabia, the proportion of palliative care needs relative to deaths has been estimated to be as high as 95% [23].

Cancer incidence in Arab countries is on the rise, and it is forecasted to increase by 1.8-fold by 2030 [24, 25]. Most of the cancer cases in Arab countries are in stage IV when treatment options are minimal, and the prognosis is usually poor, especially among young patients [26]. Traditionally, palliative care is introduced late in oncology, often when treatment options are exhausted or when death is imminent [27]. However, evidence increasingly supports integrating early palliative care into oncology practice to manage symptoms and align treatment plans with patients' value goals [27–30]. Despite these benefits, many terminally ill patients worldwide remain underserved, and referrals to interdisciplinary palliative care remain limited [1, 30].

3.1 Overview of existing palliative care in the Arab world

Palliative care is considered a new specialty in medicine and is in the early stages across the Arab World [31]. In the Middle East, palliative care is still a relatively new concept. It was first introduced in Saudi Arabia in 1992 and has only recently been adopted in countries like Qatar, Bahrain, and the UAE. The Worldwide Hospice Palliative Care Alliance (WHPCA) classified palliative care development into four levels according to the development of the services. Counties included in Level 1 are those with no hospice or palliative care activity reported. Level 2 countries have initiated capacity-building activity in palliative care, while those with isolated or generalized palliative care services are categorized as Level 3. If the government has palliative care services integrated into mainstream service provision, it will be classified as Level 4. Level 4a is for preliminary integration, and Level 4b is for advanced integration. While most Middle Eastern countries, including Palestine, Iraq, Oman, and Lebanon, are still in capacity-building, Saudi Arabia and Jordan have already established localized provisions, leading by example without integration with mainstream service providers. However, Yemen and Syria have little to no known palliative care activity. Common factors hindering progress in most countries include political issues, resource scarcity, and a lack of education and awareness [32, 33].

Despite the progress in the Arab world, no Arab country has yet reached level 4, where palliative care is fully integrated into national healthcare systems. The current Palliative Care Programs in these countries aim primarily to provide palliative care to cancer patients, including pain and symptom management. These programs sometimes support other terminal illnesses, such as non-malignant conditions (**Table 1**). However, here are some examples of initiatives and progress aiming to level up palliative care in Arab countries: Saudi Arabia has incorporated palliative care into its Healthcare Vision 2030, recognizing its importance for improving patients' outcomes [34]. The King Hussein Cancer Centre (KHCC) in Jordan is considered a comprehensive cancer center, offering well-developed palliative care for cancer patients inpatients, outpatient, and home-based care [35, 36]. In Lebanon, the Balsam Organization (a non-governmental organization) supports patients with life-threatening illnesses through clinical care, advocacy, capacity-building efforts, and research [37]. Non-government organizations, such as the Al Malath organization in Jordon, provide hospice care, addressing gaps in formal palliative care infrastructure [38].

While such initiatives are promising, the absence of national palliative care programs in many countries highlights persistent challenges. Limited resources

Level of palliative care development	Countries
Level 1—no known palliative care activity	Comoros, South Sudan, Djibouti, Iraq, Somalia, Somaliland, Syria, Yemen
Level 2—capacity building palliative care activity	UAE
Level 3a—isolate palliative care provision	Algeria, Mauritania, Bahrain, Egypt, Kuwait, Lebanon, Libya, Morocco, Palestine, Sudan, Tunisia
Level 3b—generalized palliative care provision	Jordan, Oman, Qatar, Saudi Arabia
Level 4a—palliative care services at the preliminary stage of integration	None
Level 4b—palliative care at an advanced stage of integration	None

Table 1.
Levels of palliative care development across Arab countries as assessed by the Worldwide Hospice Palliative Care Alliance (WHPCA) [32].

and cultural misconceptions surrounding palliative care require national strategies, capacity-building programs, and cultural advocacy to address barriers [31]. By integrating palliative care into healthcare systems, Arab countries can ensure holistic patient-centered care that improves the quality of life of terminally ill patients and their families.

3.2 Pediatric palliative care

In 2019, the estimated number of children requiring palliative care in the Gulf Cooperation Council (GCC) was approximately 22,000, translating to a rate of 17.5 per 10,000 children. Oman reported the highest ratio (21 per 10,000 children), while the United Arab Emirates reported the lowest (16 per 10,000 children) [39, 40]. According to the WHO, all GCC countries share health system disadvantages, including disorganized infrastructure, weak policy development, and limited regulatory capacity [39, 40].

In GCC countries, pediatric palliative care (PPC) remains underdeveloped, with services primarily catering to adults. Among the GCC nations, evidence of PPC provision exists only in Kuwait and Saudi Arabia, according to the International Children's Palliative Care Network (ICPCN) [39]. The remaining GCC countries lack specialized PPC services. This underdevelopment is further mirrored across the Middle East, where PPC is in its infancy, due to several barriers, including inadequate professional training, insufficient policymaker support, restricted access to opioids, and limited financial resources. Specialized PPC services exist only in Jordan, Egypt, and Saudi Arabia, leaving the broader region underserved [39, 40].

3.3 Availability and accessibility

Palliative care services in Arab countries are not evenly distributed, and in many cases, there are challenges for patients to access, especially for rural, remote, and marginalized populations [41]. Existing services are primarily concentrated in big cities, often within tertiary hospitals or cancer centers, limiting outreach and accessibility [41]. This urban-centric model excludes significant portions of the population, particularly those in underserved areas [41, 42]. Structural health system challenges, including poor referral systems, limited human resources, and inadequate infrastructure, further compound the situation. For instance, most palliative care facilities are hospital-based and designed for acute, curative care, leading to overcrowding and suboptimal patient experiences. Transportation difficulties and the absence of well-coordinated referral networks exacerbate the strain on families seeking care [42, 43]. Additionally, while some country-specific studies offer valuable insights into PPC service availability and gaps, such studies are scarce across the region. General reports and surveys often lack granularity, failing to address the specific needs of local populations. This insufficiency highlights the urgent need for strategic planning, standardized training programs, and integrated care frameworks that enhance the reach and quality of palliative care.

3.4 Challenges in providing palliative care in Arab countries

3.4.1 Policies and regulations barriers

Arab countries face substantial healthcare system challenges, exacerbated by insufficient funding, limited health insurance coverage, constrained resource allocation, and a shortage of healthcare professionals. Furthermore, there is an almost complete reliance on government services as the primary source of budget allocations, further complicating the situation. However, context-specific indicators are an excellent source for assessing the development of palliative care in Arab countries. Some of these indicators are related to opioid consumption and availability [44].

Opioid consumption in the Arab world is significantly lower than international recommendations and averages, with considerable variations between countries. The average usage in the region is 2.40 mg per capita per year, much lower than the 200 mg per capita per year, which is considered adequate for medical purposes [42]. Morphine, in oral and injectable forms, is predominantly available in certain countries such as Qatar, Saudi Arabia, Oman, Kuwait, Jordan, and Palestine. In contrast, other countries like Egypt and Morocco show inconsistent availability, with injectable morphine being accessible only sporadically. However, these differences from global use were not subjected to further studies to understand the core issues related to the reduced amount used, apart from a restrained supply (**Figure 2**) [44].

The bar graph illustrates opioid consumption per capita (mg/capita/year) in selected Arab countries compared to the global average of 200 mg/capita/year. Each orange bar represents a specific Arab country, while the red-dashed line highlights the global average. The graph reveals a significant disparity, with all Arab countries reporting opioid consumption well below the international benchmark. For instance, Jordan and Kuwait show relatively higher values (7 and 6 mg, respectively), while countries like Egypt and Morocco report even lower levels (2.8 and 2.5 mg).

This stark difference underscores systemic challenges, including stigma surrounding opioid use, restricted availability, and regulatory barriers, which hinder effective pain management in palliative care settings. Addressing these disparities is crucial for improving the quality of life for patients with life-limiting illnesses.

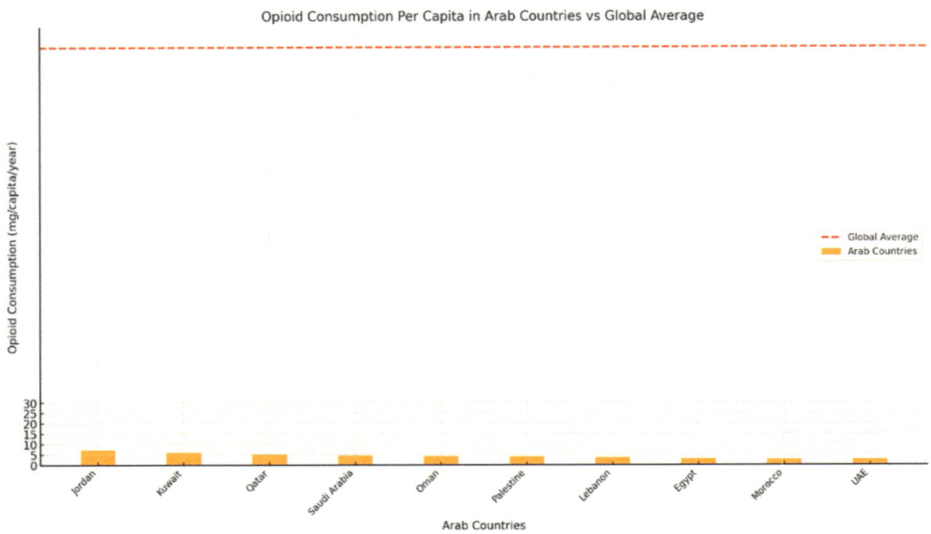

Figure 2.
Opioid consumption per capita (mg/capita/year) in selected Arab countries compared to the global average of 200 mg/capita/year.

3.4.2 Palliative care policies and funding

National strategic plans exist in Jordan, Kuwait, Lebanon, Oman, Qatar, and Saudi Arabia, and periodic evaluations are conducted in Kuwait, Qatar, and Saudi Arabia. National regulations related to Do Not Attempt Resuscitation (DNAR) policies are reported in only five countries: Lebanon, Jordan, Saudi Arabia, Qatar, and Oman [24]. Funding for palliative care is generally limited and often embedded within national cancer care plans, highlighting the need for expanded financial commitment [44].

3.4.3 Capacity building

Investing in education and workforce development is vital for addressing the shortage of palliative care professionals. Key strategies include expanding medical schools, creating specialized training programs, and providing attractive incentives for healthcare professionals to practice in understaffed regions. Integrating palliative care education into undergraduate and postgraduate medical curricula is critical.

3.5 Challenges in providing palliative care

3.5.1 Integration of palliative care services

A significant barrier to quality palliative care in Arab countries is the lack of integration into existing healthcare systems. As a result, referral to palliative care services is often delayed, leading to prolonged suffering and reduced quality of life for patients and their family members [34].

3.5.2 Lack of knowledge

A critical challenge stems from insufficient awareness of palliative care among the general public, patients, and professionals. The term "palliative" is often misinterpreted as synonymous with abandonment or treatment failure, creating resistance to its use. This leads to fear or denial of service by patients and their families and results in healthcare professionals delaying referrals, believing it signals giving up hope. To counter this, open communication and education are vital. Healthcare providers must emphasize that palliative care aims to alleviate suffering, optimize well-being, and support patients in decision-making. Palliative care is not about giving up but ensuring comfort, dignity, and quality of life. Challenging these misperceptions will foster a culture of acceptance and early referrals to palliative services [1, 45].

3.5.3 Location of care

Palliative care services in Arab countries are predominantly hospital-based, which does not align with many patients' preferences to receive care at home or in community settings. It is essential to broaden the accessibility and availability of palliative care by integrating it into various settings, such as home-based care, community centers, and outpatient clinics. By diversifying the delivery of palliative care, we can better meet the preferences and needs of patients, allowing them to receive care in settings that are comforting and familiar to them.

Addressing the barriers to quality palliative care in the Arab world requires a multi-faceted approach. This includes integrating palliative care into healthcare systems, educating the public and healthcare professionals, challenging misconceptions, promoting early referral, fostering open communication, and expanding available care options. By doing so, we can ensure that all individuals facing life-limiting illnesses receive the compassionate and comprehensive care they deserve, regardless of their location or circumstances [46].

3.5.4 Policies and regulations barriers

Systemic barriers, such as inadequate policies and regulatory frameworks, hinder palliative care's comprehensive implementation and modernization. Key challenges are limited access to controlled medications (e.g., opioids) and the absence of national policies supporting palliative care as a standard service. Therefore, reforming healthcare policies requires stakeholders' and government support, access to evidence-based and cost-effective palliative care services, and early integration of palliative care. Palliative care should be available right from the moment of diagnosis, that is, early integration, allowing a continuum of care throughout the patient's journey [45–51].

3.6 Socioeconomic factors affecting access

Arab countries vary considerably in per capita gross national income, which is a key measure for determining the extent of available resources for healthcare. It is worth noting that several countries in this region exhibit below-average healthcare spending, contributing to the world's most significant discrepancies in health expenditure. Consequently, they face a disproportionate burden of ill health stemming from numerous public health challenges, including an alarmingly high incidence of non-communicable diseases [46].

3.7 Training and education

Training and education of healthcare providers in palliative care services are crucial and indispensable for achieving the desired outcomes. It is essential that undergraduate education not only covers the fundamental principles but also provides clear and in-depth knowledge and understanding of the complex aspects of care, emphasizing its significant impact on patients entering the final stages of their lives. Unfortunately, it is disheartening to see that most Arab nations currently lack undergraduate education in the field of palliative care, thereby depriving future healthcare providers of the critical knowledge and skills necessary for effective service.

Six Arab countries have responded differently regarding the presence of official specialization programs in palliative medicine. Lebanon designates Palliative Care as a specialty; Qatar, Jordan, and Saudi Arabia as a sub-specialty; Iraq, Kuwait, and the Occupied Palestinian Territories officially recognize specializations completed abroad [44]. The King Hussain Cancer Foundation and The Saudi Society of Palliative Care have established two-year fellowship training programs in Jordan and Saudi Arabia. These specialized palliative services, operating from Cancer and Central Hospitals, have been developed through comprehensive curriculum development and rigorous fellowship programs to prepare practice specialists. These efforts reflect a positive and encouraging trend toward enhancing the overall quality of palliative care in the Arab region [34, 47].

3.8 Recommendations and future directions

Healthcare systems serving Arab and Muslim patients must address cultural and religious barriers to improve palliative care delivery. Recommendations include providing education for healthcare providers on cultural competency and the specific needs of Muslim patients, including religious practices related to end-of-life care, encouraging community engagement to dispel myths about palliative care and opioid use through public awareness campaigns, incorporating multidisciplinary teams, including spiritual advisors and culturally trained social workers, to address the holistic needs of patients and families (**Table 2**) [12, 13].

Category	Recommendation	Goal
Short-term goals	Increase public awareness through media campaigns	Raising awareness and acceptance of palliative care.
	Provide training workshops for healthcare professionals	Improving healthcare professionals' knowledge and skills.
Long-term goals	Establish national palliative care programs	Creating sustainable, formalized care systems.
	Integrate services into all levels of healthcare.	Ensuring palliative care is widely accessible and embedded in healthcare systems.

Table 2.
Future directions and recommendations for enhancing palliative care in the Arab world.

4. Psychosocial complexity in palliative care in Arabs societies

4.1 Understanding psychosocial aspects of patient and family care

4.1.1 The psychological impact of terminal illness

Patients with advanced disease or who are approaching death may experience several psychological symptoms that may exacerbate their suffering. One of the most common of these mental health problems faced by terminally ill patients is depression, affecting around 20% of individuals [52, 53]. These patients struggle to find pleasure and meaning in their final days, experiencing a sense of isolation or brokenness. These challenges of loss not only devastate the patient but also concurrently affect their families and loved ones around them. These include grievances for changes to social and occupational status, changes in role definition, loss of identity, reduced control of day-to-day activities, and physical losses experienced by the illness, also coined as anticipatory grief [54, 55]. In these patients, there lies difficulty for clinicians to differentiate between a normal emotional response to dying compared to more clinical psychiatric disorders such as major depression, leading to underdiagnosis and undertreatment [52].

Additionally, patients receiving palliative treatment also experience heightened anxiety, with around 14% meeting the cutoff range for anxiety disorders. A scoping review of qualitative studies assessing the psychosocial impact of advanced disease progression identified themes of uncertainty, worrying about the emotional impact of the disease progression on their loved ones, and fear of death, among other themes that lead to heightened anxiety [56]. In the Middle East, research has shown similar psychological impacts that are compounded by cultural factors, where terminally ill patients in the Middle East often experience the same psychological distress exacerbated by societal expectations and family dynamics [57]. Long-term psychological distress in this population may lead to a reduced quality of life for the patient and their families and difficulties with treatment adherence that may result in a strain on services [55, 58].

4.2 Coping mechanisms among patients and families

Despite the psychological burden caused by terminal illness on patients and families, various coping mechanisms can be effective in managing some of the distress, where they have been shown to improve the quality of life and depressive symptoms for both patients and their families [59]. Positive or adaptive coping strategies include active coping, acceptance, positive reframing, planning, and humor. These strategies are associated with increased resilience and reduced emotional distress. Conversely, negative coping strategies such as behavioral disengagement, self-blame, and denial are linked to increased emotional distress and decreased resilience [60].

Social support from family, friends, and healthcare professionals plays a crucial role in helping patients and their families cope with the challenges of terminal illness. Social support effectively alleviates psychological distress, providing individuals with security and belonging. Another aspect of coping can be facilitated when conserving the dignity of patients, which is a fundamental goal in palliative care [58]. In the Middle East, the concept of dignity is understood differently from the Western perspective, influenced by social, political, and cultural factors. Factors that enhance dignity include maintaining privacy, gentle communication, family support, and access to quality healthcare [61].

Culture and religion play a pivotal role in shaping the responses of patients and their families to terminal illnesses in non-Eurocentric cultures. Faith and prayer are common means of finding comfort and meaning, with religion as a significant source of psychological support [62]. Cultural traditions emphasize the importance of family and social support, enhancing individuals' ability to cope with psychological stress.

4.3 Role of cultural beliefs in psychosocial support

Cultural beliefs shape how patients and their families perceive and engage with palliative care services. Cultural norms and religious values often influence decisions about end-of-life care. For instance, the importance of family involvement and the collective decision-making process is deeply rooted in many non-Eurocentric cultures. This can affect how psychosocial support is provided and received, as healthcare providers must navigate these cultural dynamics to offer adequate care.

4.4 Stigma and misconceptions about palliative care

Despite the extensive evidence base showing the importance of early integration of palliative care in advanced cancer, there is a stigma around the discipline that remains. Additionally, the psychosocial complexity in palliative care is significantly influenced by cultural beliefs and societal attitudes, which can vary widely across different regions or cultural backgrounds. One of the significant challenges in providing palliative care in these regions is the stigma and misconceptions associated with it. Many people equate palliative care with giving up on treatment or see it as only relevant at the very end of life. This misconception can prevent patients from seeking timely palliative care designed to improve the quality of life at any stage of the illness [63]. As a result of this stigma, many physicians may also tend to avoid making timely referrals to palliative care out of fear that it would emphasize the thought of death and reduce hope or evoke negative emotions for patients and their families [64].

The stigma surrounding palliative care can lead to delays in accessing necessary services, resulting in unmanaged symptoms and reduced quality of life. Patients and families may avoid discussing palliative care options due to fear of being perceived as hopeless or giving up. This stigma is often compounded by a lack of awareness and understanding of what palliative care entails [65]. As a result, there is an emphasis on better education and awareness to combat these stigmas (**Table 3**).

4.5 The importance of culturally sensitive communication

Within the palliative care context, the role of culture is significantly acknowledged, as it is believed to facilitate how illness is understood, how suffering and pain are expressed, and how grief presents itself for the patient and their families [66]. As such, preferences in communication patterns are integral for clinicians to understand when working within this context. These differences may include a patient's preferences about knowing the extent of details of their illness, inappropriate and appropriate terminology, and levels of family involvement. For example, some culture's view talking about death as hastening the process and prefer not to name death during communication [67]. Another example includes how suffering and physical pain are recognized to be an examination of faith for some black Caribbean experiencing cancer and should not be alleviated with medications [68]. Clinicians can be mindful of these processes by inquiring about how much the individual knows and wishes to

Barrier	Impact	Proposed solution
Stigma around opioids	Underutilization of pain relief	Education campaigns debunking myths
Lack of training for professionals	Suboptimal patient care	Integrating palliative care into medical curricula
Poor access to services	Limited care for rural populations	Expanding home-based care programs

Table 3.
Overview of key barriers to adequate palliative care, their associated impacts, and proposed solutions.

know about their illness and be curious about the cultural context of their meanings of suffering, as this would influence their decision-making process [69].

Jibeen and Khalid [70] explored the acculturative stress experienced by Pakistani immigrant adolescents in Canada. They highlight that culturally sensitive communication can significantly reduce stress by providing a supportive environment that understands immigrants' challenges in a new cultural setting. The study developed a scale to measure acculturative stress, finding that effective communication acknowledging cultural differences can help mitigate the adverse effects of acculturation, such as feelings of isolation and identity conflict. Other studies also highlighted that effective communication that respects cultural values and beliefs helps reduce conflicts between patients, families, and professionals, improving the quality of care [68]. Ensuring culturally sensitive communication is essential in maintaining trust and a collaborative relationship between professionals, patients, and their family members in palliative care settings.

4.6 Integration of psychosocial support in palliative care practices

Integrating psychosocial support in palliative care practices is a crucial aspect that significantly enhances the quality of life for patients facing life-limiting illnesses. The global development of palliative care has increasingly recognized the importance of addressing patients' physical, emotional, and psychological needs. They highlight that comprehensive palliative care, which includes psychosocial support, can alleviate the emotional distress experienced by patients and their families during end-of-life care [71].

In palliative care settings, cognitive behavioral-based interventions, acceptance and commitment therapy, meaning-based interventions, mindfulness-based interventions, and arts-based therapies are some of the commonly facilitated psychotherapeutic interventions. When addressing social stressors in these contexts, end-of-life discussion, social support interventions, and promoting advanced care planning are all integral alongside therapeutic interventions [72]. In a systematic review and meta-analysis, Warth and colleagues (2019) showed that brief psychosocial intervention, including life review techniques that aim to strengthen the individual's identity by providing them the space to reflect on essential parts of their life and music therapy, was effective in improving quality of life in palliative care patients. The data showed a reduction in both emotional and existential distress in comparison to control groups who were either on a waitlist, received no treatment, or were provided with standard care [73]. Additionally, therapeutic interventions that target death anxiety through facilitating meaning and dignity, exploring relationships, and emphasizing spiritual well-being are beneficial for patients experiencing death anxiety as a result of advanced cancer [74].

The main elements of psychotherapy in end-of-life care include a strong therapeutic alliance with the patient, where the therapist demonstrates empathy and unconditional positive regard for the patient and their experiences. Therapists should also consider adaptations needed for patients in these settings, such as reduced session time, more rescheduling, and seeing patients in less conventional settings [56].

In a systematic review exploring the integration of palliative care and psychiatry, Shalev and colleagues' [75] findings underscore the vital role of psychosocial support in managing symptoms such as depression and anxiety, suggesting that healthcare providers should be trained to deliver psychosocial interventions effectively. These interventions can include counseling, support groups, and stress management techniques, which help patients cope with their emotional challenges. By addressing these psychological aspects, palliative care can significantly improve patients' overall well-being and quality of life. This holistic approach ensures that patients receive compassionate care that respects their dignity and provides comfort in their final days [75].

5. Strategies for enhancing cultural acceptance in Arabs

5.1 Community engagement and education

5.1.1 Raising awareness about palliative care

One of the challenges in integrating palliative care into patient treatment is the lack of patient awareness about it. This issue stems from inadequate resources for educating patients and the absence of detailed information outlining the specific aspects of palliative care, resulting in insufficient evidence of patient awareness [76]. A study in Jordan using the "Palliative Care Knowledge Scale" (PaCKS) and the "Frommelt Attitudes Toward Care of the Dying - B (FATCOD-B)" tool revealed moderate knowledge and neutral attitudes toward palliative care among 329 adult respondents. Only 20.4% had prior knowledge of palliative care, with higher self-reported knowledge, older age, and higher income associated with better understanding and more favorable attitudes. These findings indicate a need for awareness campaigns to educate the Jordanian society about palliative care [77].

Raising awareness is vital for integrating palliative care into public health. Campaigns should balance short-term national media efforts with long-term local initiatives. National and regional projects must address barriers such as literacy and resource access [78]. Public awareness of palliative care services is insufficient, and many families lack experience with them. Campaigns are needed to enhance awareness and improve access to these services [79].

A systematic review found that over half of the patients lacked information about palliative or hospice care. Some patients had accurate definitions, while others had misconceptions. The review recommended video presentations and community information distribution to increase awareness, emphasizing the need for patient education programs and interventional studies [76].

Some studies have shown that palliative care services are inaccessible or underdeveloped in many regions worldwide. It is emphasized that one of the key steps to introducing or developing palliative care services is to enhance awareness and community participation. This can be achieved through various awareness modalities and campaigns such as social media campaigns, national palliative care day events, and gatherings to share personal stories to foster a discussion on palliative care, such as the "human library" initiative. Additionally, community participation can be enhanced through volunteering programs like the "Adopt a Grandma" initiative and medical student-led projects [80]. The community plays a crucial role and must be included in plans to develop palliative care services. Promoting palliative care education and certification for physicians and nurses is vital, and home-based and hospice services must be maintained [81].

Palliative care is still a relatively new concept in the Middle East. Common factors hindering progress in most countries include political issues, resource scarcity, and a lack of education and awareness [33]. Recently, a strong focus has been on providing formal education to professionals and increasing public awareness. Cross-border collaborations are also essential, whether through organizations like the Middle East Cancer Consortium (MECC) or other means [33]. Given the importance of palliative care services to the well-being of patients and their families, continuous training activities that can overcome geopolitical challenges and change the attitudes of regulators, medical administrators, medical staff, and the public should be focused on [41].

5.1.2 Involvement of community leaders and religious figures

In most Middle Eastern countries, Islam is the predominant religion, but there are varying levels of acceptance regarding cancer, starting from diagnosis to treatment planning. Several factors shape people's attitudes toward cancer, including faith, beliefs, societal traditions, cultural taboos, and stigmas. Healthcare professionals must respect these practices and find ways to address their patients' sensitivities, thereby preserving their dignity and faith [82].

Therefore, physicians, nurses, and social workers should inquire about the patient's spiritual beliefs compassionately and respectfully. If medical science is presented as the sole solution to human suffering, patients and their families might perceive future promises as current realities. They may unfairly blame the oncologist if treatment fails. Thus, physicians must discuss the promises of medical science and its limitations [83]. A physician who understands their patient's cultural background gains an additional perspective on their situation. This understanding helps form stronger bonds, enabling the physician to better guide the patient's choices in finding meaning in their experience of suffering and death [83]. In culturally sensitive societies, such as those in Islamic countries, incorporating cultural components allows a deeper understanding of patients' lifestyles, values, norms, and expectations [83].

Without this understanding, clinicians would struggle to provide meaningful support to patients and their families, making it challenging to navigate cancer trajectories with less suffering. Therefore, clinicians must focus on healing and curing within the diverse cultural backgrounds of patients and healthcare providers. Unlike many Western societies, Islamic societies are more accepting of death and coexist with the awareness of its inevitability. This perspective influences how patients and their families view death and what lies beyond it [83]. To provide effective, culturally appropriate care to terminally ill Muslim patients, it is essential to perform Islamic rituals in a manner that acknowledges and respects the cultural differences of this population [84].

A study aimed at increasing awareness about the importance of advanced care planning and improving knowledge among healthcare providers and the public successfully engaged around 100 participants. The attendees, which included community members, healthcare professionals, medical students, and faith leaders, provided positive feedback, with over 90% rating the event as very good or excellent. The event increased awareness about advanced care planning within the Islamic community and helped healthcare providers gain insights into Islamic perspectives on the topic. This engagement model between the community and healthcare providers could also benefit other faith groups looking to discuss advanced care planning within their religious and cultural contexts [85, 86].

One example of the involvement of religious leaders in Palliative care in Oman was in the first Islamic medical meeting, where General Mufee gave a clear role in labeling terminally ill patients with a Do Not Resuscitate order. That meeting had a significant contribution to avoiding unnecessary suffering for terminally ill patients [87]. Islamic scholars generally agree that a DNR order is permissible under certain conditions. If further medical treatment is futile and the patient or their immediate relatives consent, it is allowed to issue a DNR order [88]. This is considered a form of medical treatment that is not obligatory but desirable (musthub). However, if the patient is not in a vegetative state and CPR could save their life, issuing a DNR order is not permissible [89].

In Arab culture, community leaders often play a crucial role, especially during challenging discussions about serious illnesses with close family members. These leaders command respect and can include tribal chiefs, elders of extended families, or even the principal of a leading school in some communities.

A specific example from my experience involved seeking the assistance of a Mosque Sheikh to help a patient with terminal cancer disclose his diagnosis to his tribe. The patient had kept his illness a secret for many years, considering the entire tribe as his extended family. He struggled with the fear of being judged for not revealing his condition earlier. Involving the Sheikh helped him come to terms with his terminal illness and provided him with peace. After each prayer, the Sheikh encouraged the community to visit the patient, offering social conjnection and spiritual support in his final months.

5.2 Training for healthcare professionals

5.2.1 Cultural competency training

Research indicates that misunderstandings between Muslim patients and non-Muslim healthcare staff are common, particularly concerning end-of-life care and pain management. Chaplains, who act as cultural and spiritual liaisons, can play a crucial role in bridging these gaps. Non-Muslim chaplains and healthcare providers should invest in deepening their understanding of Islamic beliefs and practices. This can foster better communication, respect, and trust, ultimately improving patient outcomes. Additionally, Muslim patients and their families could greatly benefit from enhanced education and awareness regarding the roles and availability of chaplains, as well as the various options for pain management and end-of-life care. These insights hold significant implications for medical practice, education, and research [90].

A study in the UAE highlighted the challenges posed by cultural diversity in adopting a holistic approach to patient care, stressing the need for culturally competent practices that respect and accommodate diverse cultural backgrounds [82]. Another study in Saudi Arabia emphasized the importance of family presence, the observance of religious practices in the absence of family, and the provision of peaceful and compassionate end-of-life experiences. These findings underline the commitment of nurses and healthcare providers to deliver holistic, patient-centered care that honors cultural and individual beliefs [91].

Healthcare institutions should implement mandatory cultural competency training programs for all providers and chaplains. These programs should cover the basics of Islamic beliefs, cultural practices, and the specific needs of Muslim patients, particularly in the context of end-of-life care and pain management. Regular workshops and seminars led by experienced Muslim chaplains and cultural experts can enhance the understanding and empathy of healthcare providers, thereby improving the overall quality of patient care.

5.2.2 Palliative care and death literacy

Death literacy refers to the knowledge and skills that enable individuals to access, understand, and make informed choices about end-of-life and death care options. It encompasses practical knowledge about good end-of-life care, the legal processes, and the support available at different stages. Death literacy prepares individuals to make informed end-of-life care decisions and support others in similar situations [92].

Despite the critical importance of death literacy, it is often inadequately addressed in medical and postgraduate education. A scoping review of death and dying education in U.S. medical schools found significant variation in the type and content of end-of-life training, with a reliance on brief, skill-based workshop interventions and limited longitudinal integration into curricula. Similarly, postgraduate education often lacks comprehensive training in death literacy, leading to a knowledge gap and comfort in end-of-life conversations [93].

Postgraduate and continuing education for palliative care professionals should emphasize training on communication techniques for addressing sensitive palliative and end-of-life topics within diverse cultural settings. Healthcare providers must be introduced, from their undergraduate education, to the importance of interprofessional collaboration when dealing with complex cross-cultural issues [94]. Encouraging healthcare providers to reflect critically on their biases and preconceptions in clinical practice can lead to more compassionate and culturally competent care [94].

A study conducted in Lebanon revealed that healthcare professionals often feel inadequately prepared to deliver palliative care, highlighting the need for enhanced education and training programs [19]. Another study in Egypt emphasized the necessity of improving healthcare providers' knowledge and attitudes toward palliative care to ensure better patient outcomes [20].

5.3 Interdisciplinary approaches to palliative care

Palliative care in Arab countries is evolving, with interdisciplinary approaches playing a crucial role in addressing the complex needs of patients with serious illnesses. These approaches involve the collaboration of various healthcare professionals, including doctors, nurses, social workers, chaplains, and other specialists, to provide comprehensive and holistic care. The World Health Organization (WHO) emphasizes integrating palliative care into primary health care (PHC). In the context of EMR countries, a tailored model is required to address their unique context [95].

A successful palliative care model requires oversight by the Ministry of Health (MOH) to guide policymaking, develop clinical guidelines, and tackle challenges in care delivery. Appointing a dedicated focal person or working group within the MOH is essential to these efforts. Key components of the model include ensuring access to necessary pain medications, facilitating their use in home settings, and providing empowerment courses for care providers to address various challenges. Establishing community movements, non-governmental organizations (NGOs), and volunteer groups are equally important. Additionally, robust monitoring and evaluation systems are vital to ensuring service quality and continuity, supported by an appropriate payment system [95].

Research plays a critical role in developing and evaluating palliative care practices through conducting needs assessment studies, providing evidence-based practice, and setting indicators to evaluate existing programs [96]. The model also prioritizes community health workers, particularly nurses, as versatile professionals in delivering community palliative care. Networking, collaboration, and integrating digital health technologies are emphasized to support nurses in this role [95].

In recent years, there has been a shift toward community-based palliative care, which aims to provide care in patients' homes and communities rather than in hospitals. This approach helps to reduce the burden on healthcare facilities and allows patients to receive care in a familiar and comfortable environment. Community-based palliative care also promotes the involvement of family members in the care process, which is highly valued in Arab cultures.

However, there are several challenges to implementing interdisciplinary palliative care in Arab countries. These include the lack of integration of palliative care into national health policies, limited interprofessional collaboration, and a shortage of trained healthcare professionals. Additionally, there is a need for increased public awareness about palliative care and its benefits.

5.4 Policy recommendations

5.4.1 Advocacy for palliative care inclusion in healthcare policies

This advocacy effort requires robust evaluation and indicator data to measure the extent of practitioner involvement in global and regional advocacy, particularly in low- and middle-income countries (LMICs). Effective advocacy necessitates directing more attention toward advocacy initiatives, researching suitable and cost-effective palliative care models for LMICs, and establishing a global community of practice. This community would empower practitioners to actively engage policymakers at all health system governance levels actively, facilitating systemic PC integration [97].

A study emphasized the need to incorporate palliative care (PC) into university curricula in Palestine as a mandatory course and establish advanced degree programs to address the shortage of PC specialists.

Strengthening academic infrastructure in this way would help build capacity in the field. Additionally, aligning healthcare policies with national laws could improve patient and family services while addressing existing challenges. Partnering with national and international organizations to secure funding could further support PC development, including enhancing access to essential medications and other resources [98].

5.4.2 Development of guidelines tailored to cultural contexts

The professional survey conducted in 1998 with 3000 South Australians revealed that while community awareness of palliative care was 52%; overall, it was significantly lower (37%) among respondents born outside Australia and the United Kingdom. The 1996 Australian Bureau of Statistics census highlighted that over 3 million Australians spoke a language other than English at home, with 17% reporting limited or no English proficiency. This emphasized the need to target over half a million individuals with culturally sensitive palliative care brochures in their native languages. In Adelaide and Melbourne, community consultations were conducted under the supervision of the Western Palliative Care Service Project. The consultations addressed sensitive cultural aspects such as communication of diagnosis and prognosis, family and community roles, attitudes toward pain relief, and taboos. In July 1999, during National Palliative Care Week, Brochures for the five major Cultural groups—Italian, Greek, Vietnamese, Chinese, and Polish—comprised 62% of the total print run; brochures in the remaining 15 languages followed in November 1999 [94].

The project was expanded to include multicultural guidelines, which are vital in addressing Australia's diverse cultural landscape. With its rich blend of customs, rituals, and values, it is critical to approach individuals with life-threatening illnesses and their families with cultural sensitivity and respect.

These guidelines were designed to support health professionals and caregivers by offering insights into unfamiliar customs and rituals. Input was gathered from individuals and organizations representing various cultural groups, although the guidelines are not exhaustive and recognize the existence of diverse perspectives. Health professionals are encouraged to seek guidance directly from patients and families to ensure their preferences and cultural needs are respected [94].

6. Conclusions

6.1 Summary of key points

This chapter explores the cultural acceptance of palliative care in Arab societies, focusing on historical, cultural, and religious influences that shape perceptions and practices of end-of-life care. It highlights the pivotal role of Islamic teachings, emphasizing the sanctity of life, compassion, and spiritual preparation for death. Historical contexts, such as pre-Islamic traditions and advancements during the Islamic Golden Age, have shaped family-centered caregiving practices, which remain central today. Current challenges to palliative care integration include stigma surrounding opioids, lack of professional training, and unequal access to services, particularly in rural areas. Despite progress in some countries like Jordan and Saudi Arabia, no Arab nation has fully integrated palliative care into its healthcare systems. The chapter also addresses psychosocial complexities, emphasizing the emotional and mental burden of terminal illnesses on patients and families and underscores the need for culturally sensitive communication, education campaigns, and policy reform.

6.2 The importance of fostering cultural acceptance for improved palliative care outcomes

Cultural acceptance is essential for improving palliative care outcomes in Arab societies, as deeply rooted beliefs, religious values, and family dynamics influence healthcare decisions. In societies where illness and suffering are viewed as spiritual tests, fostering cultural understanding helps dismantle misconceptions that may hinder the acceptance of palliative care interventions, such as pain management using opioids. Family collectivism, while a source of strength, can sometimes delay discussions about prognosis and treatment, underscoring the need for sensitive communication strategies. By fostering cultural acceptance through targeted education campaigns, collaboration with religious and community leaders, and integrating spiritual care into palliative practices, healthcare providers can build trust, ensure patient dignity, and address barriers to care. Embracing cultural values will enhance patients' quality of life and empower families to participate meaningfully in care decisions.

6.3 Future directions for research and practice

Research and scientific work in Arab countries has grown significantly in quantity, visibility, and impact in recent years. Nonetheless, there is limited published evidence on nursing and palliative care in these countries. In addition, most research has been conducted in collaboration with countries outside the Arab world. Future studies should prioritize building local evidence by assessing culturally tailored interventions to improve palliative care access, awareness, and delivery. Another critical area of research is exploring how to balance collective family values with patient autonomy in a culturally sensitive manner to improve decision-making in palliative settings.

For practice, emphasis should be placed on expanding palliative care training for healthcare professionals, particularly in underserved areas, and developing national policies that recognize palliative care as a standard component of healthcare. Initiatives to improve opioid accessibility, expand home-based care models, and implement early palliative care integration will be essential to ensuring equitable, high-quality care across the region. Additionally, research on integrating psychosocial support and spiritual care in palliative settings will address the emotional and mental health needs of patients and families, further aligning care practices with the cultural and religious values of Arab societies.

Acknowledgements

We thank Sultan Qaboos Comprehensive Cancer Care and Research Center and the University Medical City for the technical support.

Authors contributions

Dr. Amna Al-Harrasi: Idea Conceptualizations, Chapter Outline, Introduction, overall chapter management, Proof readings, Tables and charts, and modifications. Revision.

Dr. Amna Al-Harrasi and Dr. Nasr Al-Riyami: Cultural Context of Palliative Care in Arab Societies.

Dr. Atika AlMusalami: Current State of Palliative Care in Arab Countries.

Dr. Rawan AlMujaini and Mrs. Entesar AlYafai: Psychosocial complexity in Palliative Care in Arab Societies.

Dr. Nawal Al Mahyijari, Dr. Amna Al-Harrasi: Strategies for Enhancing Cultural Acceptance in Arabs.

Dr. Adhari AL Zaabi: Conclusions, Chapter Management and Proof Readings and Revision.

Conflict of interest

The authors have no conflict of interest to declare.

Notes/thanks/other declarations

No other declarations.

Author details

Amna Al-Harrasi[1*], Nasr Al-Riyami[1], Atika AlMusalami[2], Rawan AlMujaini[1], Entesar AlYafai[1], Nawal Al Mahyijari[1] and Adhari Al Zaabi[3]

1 Sultan Qaboos Comprehensive Cancer Care and Research Center, University Medical City, Muscat-Oman

2 National Oncology Center, Royal Hospital, Ministry of Health, Muscat-Oman

3 College of Medicine, Sultan Qaboos University, Muscat-Oman

*Address all correspondence to: a.alharrasi-2@cccrc.gov.om

References

[1] World Health Organization. WHO Definition of Palliative Care [Internet]. Geneva: WHO; 2019. Available from: https://www.who.int/cancer/palliative/definition/en/

[2] National Coalition for Hospice and Palliative Care. National Consensus Project for Quality Palliative Care Clinical Practice Guidelines. [Internet]. 2018. Richmond, VA: National Coalition for Hospice and Palliative Care. Available from: https://www.nationalcoalitionhpc.org/ncp-guidelines/ [Accessed: February 28, 2025]

[3] Kirmayer LJ, Gómez-Carrillo A. Culturally responsive clinical psychology and psychiatry: An ecosocial approach. In: Maercker A, Heim E, Kirmayer LJ, editors. Cultural clinical psychology and PTSD. Hogrefe; 2019:3-21

[4] Aoun SM, Rumbold B, Howting D, Bolleter A, Breen LJ. Bereavement support for family caregivers: The gap between guidelines and practice in palliative care. PLOS ONE. 2021;**12**(10):e0184750. DOI: 10.1371/journal.pone.0184750

[5] Rodin G, Lo C, Rydall A, Shnall J, Malfitano C, Chiu A, et al. Managing Cancer and Living Meaningfully (CALM): A randomized controlled trial of a psychological intervention for patients with advanced cancer. Journal of Clinical Oncology. 2018;**36**(23):2422-2432. DOI: 10.1200/JCO.2017.77.1097

[6] Pakenham K, Martin CL. Psychosocial palliative care: Patients' preferred intervention medium, target domains, and well-being priorities. Palliative and Supportive Care. 2024;**22**(4):742-750. DOI: 10.1017/S1478951522001535

[7] Al-Ghazi SA. End-of-life Care in Islamic Contexts: A historical perspective. Journal of Islamic Studies. 2018;**29**(2):213-231

[8] Bouhlel S. The role of family in Arab societies: Implications for palliative care. Middle Eastern Journal of Palliative Medicine. 2020;**12**(1):34-45

[9] Kamoun S, Al-Rashidi M. Palliative Care in the Muslim World: Practices and challenges. Global Health Review. 2019;**10**(3):102-115

[10] Qari M. Historical development of palliative Care in the Arab World. Arab Medical Journal. 2017;**22**(2):145-160

[11] Saba F. Family-centered palliative care in Arab societies. Journal of Family Health. 2020;**14**(2):67-75

[12] Omar S, Mohammad Z Al-Shahri, Gassan A. Culture and Spiritually Sensitive Palliative Care of Muslims with guests. Yale Cancer Center. 25 October 2015 Yale http://www.yalecancercenter.org

[13] Palliative Medicine Grand Rounds. Muslim Traditions for Patient Care at end of Life. Rochester, MN: Mayo Clinic; 2019. Available from: https://ce.mayo.edu

[14] Mukherjee A. Cultural and religious factors influencing palliative care. Journal of Palliative Care Studies. 2021;**15**(4):178-189

[15] Saad R, Al-Yousef H. Islamic perspectives on pain Management at the end of life. Pain Management and Palliative Care. 2019;**18**(2):88-97

[16] Al-Awamer A, Downar J. Developing a palliative care service model for Muslim Middle Eastern countries. Support Care Cancer. 2014;**22**(12):3253-3262. DOI: 10.1007/s00520-014-2347-4

[17] Givler A, Bhatt H, Maani-Fogelman PA. The importance of cultural competence in pain and palliative care. In: StatPearls [Internet]. Treasure Island (FL): StatPearls Publishing; 2023

[18] Glyn-Blanco MB, Lucchetti G, Badanta B. How do cultural factors influence the provision of end-of-life care? A narrative review. Applied Nursing Research. 2023;**73**:151720. ISSN 0897-1897. DOI: 10.1016/j.apnr.2023.151720

[19] Sameh E, Ayumi I, Noriko Y-M. Palliative and end-of-life care in Egypt: Overview and recommendations for improvement. International Journal of Palliative Nursing. 2020;**26**(6):284-291. DOI: 10.12968/IJPN.2020.26.6.284

[20] Leong M, Olnick S, Akmal T, Copenhaver A, Razzak R. How Islam influences end-of-life care: Education for palliative care clinicians. Journal of Pain and Symptom Management. 2016;**52**(6):771-774.e3. DOI: 10.1016/j.jpainsymman.2016.05.034

[21] Kamali MH. The Dignity of Man: An Islamic Perspective. Cambridge: Islamic Texts Society; 2002

[22] Gafer N, Gebre N, Jabeen I, et al. A model for integrating palliative care into eastern Mediterranean health systems with a primary care approach. BMC Palliative Care. 2024;**23**:264. DOI: 10.1186/s12904-024-01590-5

[23] Almobarak F. Unlocking compassion: Expanding access to palliative care in Saudi Arabia. Palliative Care & Social Practice. 2024;**18**:26323524241290828. DOI: 10.1177/26323524241290828

[24] Al-Muftah M, Al-Ejeh F. Cancer incidence and mortality estimates in Arab countries in 2018: A GLOBOCAN data analysis. Cancer Epidemiology, Biomarkers & Prevention. 2023;**32**(12):1738-1746. DOI: 10.1158/1055-9965.EPI-23-0520

[25] AlZaabi A, AlHarrasi A, AlMusalami A, AlMahyijari N, Al Hinai K, ALAdawi H, et al. Early onset colorectal cancer: Challenges across the cancer care continuum. Annals of Medicine and Surgery. 2022;**82**:104453. DOI: 10.1016/j.amsu.2022.104453

[26] Osman H, Yamout R. Palliative care in the Arab world. In: Al-Shamsi HO, Abu-Gheida IH, Iqbal F, Al-Awadhi A, editors. Cancer in the Arab World. Singapore: Springer; 2022. DOI: 10.1007/978-981-16-7945-2_24

[27] Temel JS, Greer JA, Muzikansky A, et al. Early palliative care for patients with metastatic non-small-cell lung cancer. The New England Journal of Medicine. 2010;**363**(8):733-742

[28] World Health Organization. Assessing National Capacity for the Prevention and Control of Noncommunicable Diseases: Report of the 2019 Global Survey. Geneva: World Health Organization; 2020. Licence: CC BY-NC-SA 3.0 IGO

[29] Davis MP, Temel JS, Balboni T, et al. A review of the trials which examine early integration of outpatient and home palliative care for patients with serious illnesses. Annals of Palliative Medicine. 2015;**4**(3):99-121

[30] Temel JS, Greer JA, El-Jawahri A, et al. Effects of early integrated palliative care in patients with lung and GI cancer: A randomized clinical trial. Journal of Clinical Oncology. 2017;**35**(8):834-841

[31] Phillips JL, Elvidge N, Currow D. Challenges and future directions of palliative care globally. In: MacLeod RD, Van den Block L, editors. Textbook of Palliative Care. Cham: Springer; 2024. DOI: 10.1007/978-3-319-31738-0_5-2

[32] Connor SR, editor. Global Atlas of Palliative Care. 2nd ed. London: World Hospice and Palliative Care Alliance; 2020. Available from: https://cdn.who.int/media/docs/default-source/integrated-health-services-(ihs)/csy/palliative-care/whpca_global_atlas_p5_digital_final.pdf?sfvrsn=1b54423a_3

[33] Zeinah GFA, Al-Kindi SG, Hassan AA. Middle East experience in palliative care. American Journal of Hospice & Palliative Medicine. 2013;**30**(1):94-99. DOI: 10.1177/1049909112439619

[34] Alshammary S, Altamimi I, Alhuqbani M, Alhumimidi A, Baaboud A, Altamimi A. Palliative care in Saudi Arabia: An updated assessment following the National Vision 2030 reforms. Journal of Palliative Medicine. 2024;**27**(5):651-657. DOI: 10.1089/jpm.2023.0519. Epub 2024 Jan 24

[35] Shamieh O, Alarjeh G, Hammad R, Payne S, Harding R, Sullivan R, et al. National palliative care strategy in a conflict-affected country: A Jordanian demonstration project. Journal of Pain and Symptom Management. 2024;**67**(5):e473-e485. DOI: 10.1016/j.jpainsymman.2023.12.018. Epub 2023 Dec 28

[36] Stjernswärd J, Foley KM, Ferris FD. Jordan palliative care initiative: A WHO demonstration project. Journal of Pain and Symptom Management. 2007;**33**(5):628-633

[37] Balsam Organization [Internet]. Available from: https://balsam-lb.org/

[38] Al Malath Foundation for Palliative Care [Internet]. Amman, Jordan: Al Malath Foundation for Palliative Care; 2025. Available from: https://al-malath.com/en/foundation/

[39] Alotaibi Q, Dighe M. Assessing the need for pediatric palliative care in the six Arab gulf cooperation council countries. Palliative Medicine Reports. 2023;**4**(1):36-40. DOI: 10.1089/pmr.2022.0037

[40] Mojen LK, Rassouli M, Eshghi P, Sari AA, Karimooi MH. Palliative care for children with cancer in the Middle East: A comparative study. Indian Journal of Palliative Care. 2017;**23**(4):379-385

[41] Silbermann M, Arnaout M, Daher M, et al. Palliative cancer care in middle eastern countries: Accomplishments and challenges. Annals of Oncology. 2012;**23**(Suppl. 3):15-28. DOI: 10.1093/annonc/mds084

[42] Scholten WK, Christensen AE, Olesen AE, Drewes AM. Quantifying the adequacy of opioid analgesic consumption globally: An updated method and early findings. American Journal of Public Health. 2019;**109**(1):52-57. DOI: 10.2105/AJPH.2018.304753

[43] Almalki N, Boyle B, O'Halloran P. What helps or hinders effective end-of-life care in adult intensive care units in Middle Eastern countries? A systematic review. BMC Palliative Care. 2024;**23**(1):87. DOI: 10.1186/s12904-024-01413-7

[44] Sánchez-Cárdenas MA, Pourghazian N, Garralda E, et al. Palliative care in the eastern Mediterranean: Comparative analysis using specific indicators. BMC Palliative Care. 2022;**21**(1):168. DOI: 10.1186/s12904-022-01047-7

[45] Zimmermann C, Wong JL, Swami N, et al. Public knowledge and attitudes concerning palliative care. BMJ Supportive & Palliative Care. 2024;**14**:e1085-e1095

[46] World Health Organization. Global Expenditure on Health: Public Spending on the Rise? Geneva: World Health Organization; 2021. Licence: CC BY-NC-SA 3.0 IGO

[47] Shamieh O, Richardson K, Abdel-Razeq H, Mansour A, Payne S. Gaining palliative medicine subspecialty recognition and fellowship accreditation in Jordan. Journal of Pain and Symptom Management. 2020;**60**(5):1003-1011. DOI: 10.1016/j.jpainsymman.2020.05.016

[48] Hawley P. Barriers to access to palliative care. Palliat Care. 2017;**10**:1178224216688887. DOI: 10.1177/1178224216688887

[49] Aregay A, O'Connor M, Stow J, Ayers N, Lee S. Perceived policy-related barriers to palliative care implementation: A qualitative descriptive study. Palliative Care and Social Practice. 2023;**17**:26323524231198542. DOI: 10.1177/26323524231198542

[50] Flieger SP, Chui K, Koch-Weser S. Lack of awareness and common misconceptions about palliative care among adults: Insights from a national survey. Journal of General Internal Medicine. 2020;**35**(7):2059-2064. DOI: 10.1007/s11606-020-05730-4

[51] Abu-Odah H, Molassiotis A, Liu J. Challenges on the provision of palliative care for patients with cancer in low- and middle-income countries: A systematic review of reviews. BMC Palliative Care. 2020;**19**(1):55. DOI: 10.1186/s12904-020-00558-5

[52] Breitbart W, Dickerman AL. Assessment and Management of Depression in Palliative Care. Wellesley, MA; 2024. UpToDate. Available from: https://www.uptodate.com/contents/assessment-and-management-of-depression-in-palliative-care?search=Assessment%20and%20Management%20of%20Depression%20in%20Palliative%20Care&source=search_result&selectedTitle=1%7E150&usage_type=default&display_rank=1 [Accessed: August 2024]

[53] Wilson KG, Lander M, Chochinov HM. Diagnosis and management of depression in palliative care. In: Chochinov HM, Breitbart W, editors. Handbook of Psychiatry in Palliative Medicine. New York: Oxford University Press; 2009

[54] Rousseau P. The losses and suffering of terminal illness. Mayo Clinic Proceedings. 2000;**75**(2):197-198

[55] Hottensen D. Anticipatory grief in patients with cancer. Clinical Journal of Oncology Nursing. 2010;**14**(1):106-107

[56] Kolsteren EE, Deuning-Smit E, Chu AK, van der Hoeven YC, Prins JB, van der Graaf WT, et al. Psychosocial aspects of living long term with advanced cancer and ongoing systemic treatment: A scoping review. Cancers. 2022;**14**(16):3889

[57] Al-Shahri MZ. Islamic theology and the principles of palliative care. Palliative & Supportive Care. 2016;**14**(6):635-640. DOI: 10.1017/S1478951516000080

[58] Kredentser MS, Chochinov HM. Psychotherapeutic considerations for patients with terminal illness. American Journal of Psychotherapy. 2020;**73**(4):137-143

[59] Greer JA, Applebaum AJ, Jacobsen JC, Temel JS, Jackson VA. Understanding and addressing the role of coping in palliative care for patients with advanced cancer. Journal of Clinical Oncology. 2020;**38**(9):915-925

[60] Shimizu Y, Hayashi A, Maeda I, Miura T, Inoue A, Takano M, et al.

Resilience and coping styles in family caregivers of terminally ill patients: A cross-sectional survey. Palliative & Supportive Care. 2024;**23**:1-8. DOI: 10/1017/S147895152400

[61] Dakessian Sailian S, Salifu Y, Saad R, Preston N. Dignity of patients with palliative needs in the Middle East: An integrative review. BMC Palliative Care. 2021;**20**:1-8. DOI: 10.1186/s12904-021-00791-6

[62] Gustafson C, Lazenby M. Assessing Muslim oncology patients' unique experiences and needs receiving palliative and end-of-life care: An integrative review. Journal of Palliative Care. 2019;**34**(1):52-61

[63] Alcalde J, Zimmermann C. Stigma about palliative care: Origins and solutions. Ecancer Medical Science. 2022;**16**:1377

[64] Bandieri E, Borelli E, Gilioli F, Bigi S, Mucciarini C, Ferrari U, et al. Stigma of palliative care among patients with advanced cancer and their caregivers on early palliative care. Cancers. 2023;**15**(14):3656

[65] Zimmermann C, Swami N, Krzyzanowska M, Leighl N, Rydall A, Rodin G, et al. Perceptions of palliative care among patients with advanced cancer and their caregivers. CMAJ : Canadian Medical Association Journal. 2016;**188**(10):E217-E227

[66] Bosma H, Apland L, Kazanjian A. Cultural conceptualizations of hospice palliative care: More similarities than differences. Palliative Medicine. 2010;**24**(5):510-522

[67] Colclough YY. Native American death taboo: Implications for health care providers. American Journal of Hospice and Palliative Medicine®. 2017;**34**(6):584-591

[68] Koffman J, Morgan M, Edmonds P, Speck P, Higginson IJ. "I know he controls cancer": The meanings of religion among black Caribbean and white British patients with advanced cancer. Social Science & Medicine. 2008;**67**(5):780-789

[69] Cain CL, Surbone A, Elk R, Kagawa-Singer M. Culture and palliative care: Preferences, communication, meaning, and mutual decision making. Journal of Pain and Symptom Management. 2018;**55**(5):1408-1419

[70] Jibeen T, Khalid R. Predictors of psychological well-being of Pakistani immigrants in Toronto, Canada. International Journal of Intercultural Relations. 2010;34(5):452-464. DOI: 10.1016/ j.ijintrel.2010.04.010

[71] Clark D, Wright M. The international observatory on end-of-life care: A global view of palliative care development. Journal of Pain and Symptom Management. 2007;**33**(5):542-546

[72] von Blanckenburg P, Leppin N. Psychological interventions in palliative care. Current Opinion in Psychiatry. 2018;**31**(5):389-395

[73] Warth M, Kessler J, Koehler F, Aguilar-Raab C, Bardenheuer HJ, Ditzen B. Brief psychosocial interventions improve patients' quality of life receiving palliative care: A systematic review and meta-analysis. Palliative Medicine. 2019;**33**(3):332-345

[74] Grossman CH, Brooker J, Michael N, Kissane D. Death anxiety interventions in patients with advanced cancer: A systematic review. Palliative Medicine. 2018;**32**(1):172-184

[75] Shalev D, Brenner K, Carlson RL, Chammas D, Levitt S, Noufi PE, et al. Palliative care psychiatry: Building

synergy across the spectrum. Current Psychiatry Reports. 2024;**26**(3):60-72

[76] Masoud B, Imane B, Naiire S. Patient awareness of palliative care: Systematic review. BMJ Supportive & Palliative Care. 2023;**13**:136-142

[77] Klitzman R, Di Sapia NG, Garbuzova E, et al. Muslim patients in the U.S. confronting challenges regarding end-of-life and palliative care: The experiences and roles of hospital chaplains. BMC Palliative Care. 2023;**22**:28. DOI: 10.1186/s12904-023-01144-1

[78] Seymour J. The impact of public health awareness campaigns on the awareness and quality of palliative care. Journal of Palliative Medicine. 2018;**21**(S1):S-30–S36

[79] McIlfatrick S, Hasson F, McLaughlin D, et al. Public awareness and attitudes toward palliative care in Northern Ireland. BMC Palliative Care. 2013;**12**:34. DOI: 10.1186/1472-684X-12-34

[80] Shahriah S, Dwivedi S, Amornmahaphun S, et al. Awareness building and improving participation of local communities in palliative care. Palliative Medicine in Practice. 2024;**18**(3):163-168

[81] Altarifi AA, Baker M, Abedal-Kareem K, et al. Knowledge and attitude of the general public toward palliative care in Jordan: A cross-sectional study. American Journal of Hospice & Palliative Medicine. 2025;**42**(1):94-101. DOI: 10.1177/10499091241231781

[82] Saleh AM, Hejase R, Abdel-Aziz HR. Unity in faith: A literature review on cultural and spiritual health interventions for cancer patients. International Journal of Africa Nursing Sciences. 2024;**20**:100768

[83] Salman K, Zoucha R. Considering faith within culture when caring for the terminally ill Muslim patient and family. Journal of Hospice and Palliative Nursing. 2010;**12**(3):156-163. DOI: 10.1097/NJH.0b013e3181d76d26

[84] Heirali AA, Javed S, Damani Z, et al. Muslim perspectives on advance care planning: A model for community engagement. Palliative Care and Social Practice. 2021;**15**. DOI: 10.1177/26323524219971 52

[85] Mani ZA. Bridging cultural gaps in end-of-life care: The experiences of international charge nurses in Saudi Arabia. BMC Nursing. 2024;**23**:865. DOI: 10.1186/s12912-024-02514-7

[86] Al-Adawi SSH, Al Lamki Z, Moustafa AA, Alkindi S, Al-Adawi S. Palliative care in a society in transition: How to address the unmet biopsychosocial needs in Oman. In: Laher I, editor. Handbook of Healthcare in the Arab World. Cham: Springer; 2021. DOI: 10.1007/978-3-030-36811-1_188

[87] Sultan Qaboos University. First Medical Islamic Meeting. Muscat, Oman: Sultan Qaboos University; 2012. Available from: https://youtu.be/gOqB8Jm5MQM [Accessed: January 18, 2025]

[88] Darul Ifta Birmingham. DNR - IslamQA. Birmingham, UK: Darul Ifta Birmingham; 2025. Available from: https://islamqa.org/hanafi/daruliftaamw/19594/dnr/ [Accessed: January 18, 2025]

[89] Darul Ifta MW. Placing a Patient under DNR (Do Not Resuscitate). IslamQA. Johannesburg, South Africa: Darul Ifta MW; 2023. Available from: https://islamqa.org/hanafi/daruliftaamw/134415/placing-a-patient-under-dnr-do-not-resuscitate/

[90] Silbermann MD, PhD HEA. Cultural perspectives in cancer care: Impact of Islamic traditions and practices in middle eastern countries. Journal of Pediatric Hematology/Oncology. 2011;**33**:S81-S86. DOI: 10.1097/MPH.0b013e318230dab6

[91] Fadhil I et al. Barriers to, and opportunities for, palliative care development in the eastern Mediterranean region. The Lancet Oncology. 2017;**18**(3):e176-e184

[92] Canberra Health Literacy. Death literacy. Available from: https://cbrhl.org.au/what-is-health-literacy/death-literacy/?form=MG0AV3 [Accessed: January 18, 2025]

[93] Patterson L, Decker A, Weaver R, Bolkan C, King A, Roman A. Death and dying education in US medical schools: A scoping review. Innovation in Aging. 2023;**7**(Suppl. 1):311. DOI: 10.1093/geroni/igad104.1034

[94] Weber O, Semlali I, Gamondi C, et al. Cultural competency and sensitivity in the curriculum for palliative care professionals: A survey in Switzerland. BMC Medical Education. 2021;**21**:318. DOI: 10.1186/s12909-021-02745-1

[95] Rosa WE, Ahmed E, Chaila MJ, Chansa A, Cordoba MA, Dowla R, et al. Can you hear us now? Equity in global advocacy for palliative care. Journal of Pain and Symptom Management. 2022;**64**(4):e217-e226

[96] Silbermann M, Fink RM, Min SJ, Mancuso MP, Brant J, Hajjar R, et al. Evaluating palliative care needs in middle eastern countries. Journal of Palliative Medicine. 2015;**18**(1):18-25. DOI: 10.1089/jpm.2014.0194

[97] Abu-Odah H, Molassiotis A, Liu JY. Gathering policymakers' perspectives as an essential step in planning and implementing palliative care services at a national level: An example from a resource-limited country. BMC Palliative Care. 2022;**21**:43. DOI: 10.1186/s12904-022-00936-1

[98] Taylor A, Box M. Multicultural Palliative Care Guidelines. Yarralumla, Australia: Palliative Care; 1999. ISBN: 0-646-38432-5